Surviving "Terminal" Cancer

SURVIVING "TERMINAL" CANCER

*Clinical Trials, Drug Cocktails, and Other Treatments
Your Oncologist Won't Tell You About*

by Ben Williams, PhD

Fairview Press • Minneapolis

Library of Congress Cataloging-in-Publication Data
Williams, Ben (Ben A.), 1944-
Surviving "terminal" cancer : clinical trials, drug cocktails, and other treatments your oncologist won't tell you about / by Ben Williams.
     p. cm.
  Includes bibliographical references and index.
     ISBN 10: 1-47749-651-3; ISBN 13: 978-1-47749-651-0
1. Williams, Ben (Ben A.), 1944---Health. 2.Brain--Cancer--Patients--United States--Biography. 3. Self-care, Health. 4. Cancer--Treatment--United States. 5. Cancer--Alternative treatment. 6. Health services accessibility--United States. I. Title.
RC280.B7 W54 2002
362.1'9699481'0992--dc21

                        2002006828

First printing: August 2002
Printed in Canada
12 11 10 09 08 07   10 9 8 7 6

Cover by Laurie Ingram

Medical Disclaimer
This publication is designed to provide accurate and authoritative information in regard to the subject matter covered. It is sold with the understanding that the publisher is not engaged in the provision or practice of medical, nursing, or professional healthcare advice or services in any jurisdiction. If medical advice or other professional assistance is required, the services of a qualified and competent professional should be sought. Fairview Press is not responsible or liable, directly or indirectly, for any form of damages whatsoever resulting from the use (or misuse) of information contained in or implied by these documents.

Fairview Press publications, including *Surviving "Terminal" Cancer,* do not necessarily reflect the philosophy of Fairview Health Services.

To Diane, who was there when I needed her

Contents

Acknowledgments

I thank Susan Herrnstein and Sadanand Singh for their suggestions after reading an early draft of this book. I also thank John Wixted, Hal Pashler, and Brett Clementz for their help in my search for an effective treatment plan.

Introduction

If I made a list of the most terrible things that could happen to someone, a malignant brain tumor would be very near the top. Any form of cancer can be devastating, but brain cancer carries its own special horror. Your brain is the foundation of your personality, your intellect, your emotions, your motor functions—the very basis of your being. As a tumor invades your neural tissue, your abilities deteriorate to the point where you can no longer function. It can be an ugly way to die.

Brain cancer is among the most malignant forms of cancer. The most common, and deadly, of brain tumors are glioblastomas (technically known as glioblastoma multiformes, or GBMs). Glioblastomas grow rapidly. Given that the brain is confined to the boundaries of the skull, it takes very little time for a glioblastoma to grow large enough to put lethal pressure on the brain. Other brain tumors are not nearly as vicious, but all eventually will be fatal unless successfully treated. There is no such thing as a good type of brain tumor.

I was diagnosed with a glioblastoma in the spring of 1995. My story, I hope, will be a model for those confronting any type of cancer, although a glioblastoma has its own unique features. Describing what I have learned while coping with this deadly disease is the purpose of this book.

Ten years ago, physicians had little to offer glioblastoma patients. The universal opinion was that anyone with a glioblastoma was certain to die from it. Some would die within three to four months, some after six to nine months, and the very lucky might survive as long as eighteen months. But all would die. The prognosis has improved somewhat over the past ten years, but hardly enough to change the eventual outcome by more than a few months. Patients still are told they have no chance of survival, and physicians' most common advice is to forgo treatment and try to make the best of the time remaining. Unfortunately, there is not much good time involved, and people who are undergoing the destruction of their brain and facing imminent death are not known for their joviality.

But this dire prognosis is contradicted by a number of case histories, including my own. There are long-term survivors of this terrible disease. Although the odds of survival remain very low, there are grounds for hope. In the near future, new and more successful treatments will become available. In the meantime, conventional medicine has its limits, and cancer patients need to explore treatment options not yet incorporated into conventional medical practice. Patients must be willing to go beyond their physicians' advice, and sometimes follow options contrary to that advice. This is not an easy road to travel. Newly diagnosed patients are confronted with a disease about which they are largely ignorant. For better or for worse, they often are at the mercy of their physicians. Some physicians will actively resist any approach to treatment other than their own, even when they concede that their treatment offers little promise. Therefore, patients need to learn how to acquire medical information on their own while exploiting their physicians' knowledge and expertise. To do both simultaneously requires considerable patience, social skill, and effort.

The current technological age offers opportunities that patients did not have ten years ago. Using the Internet, it is now possible to find medical information quickly, and to exchange advice and treatment information with patients around the world. Access to information allows patients to take a more active approach in determining their treatment. While this may be disconcerting to some physicians, it greatly improves patient outcome. New medical treatments are appearing at an unprecedented pace, and it is essential to be on the cutting edge. Patients whose physicians are only a few years behind may miss potentially life-saving treatments.

While my story is idiosyncratic, it has much in common with that of others who have been diagnosed with a deadly form of cancer. All of us hope to confront death with dignity and without fear of pain, even while doing our best to postpone the end of our lives. Observing others who have faced a similar experience provides not only solace, but insight into how best to deal with our own disease. Like soldiers going into battle, we gain strength and courage by witnessing the successful coping strategies of fellow cancer patients. This can serve as a bulwark against self-pity and depression, which can be as debilitating as the disease itself.

This book is divided into three parts. The first is a narrative of my experiences as a patient, describing the resources I marshaled while trying to cope. The second is a more general discussion of how the current medical system operates, with special emphasis on the field of oncology. Much of this section provides a harsh critique of medical conventions that serve primarily the physician and not the patient. Despite America's reputation for having the best cancer treatments available, many people are surprised and dismayed by the limited options provided by the current system, how little respect it shows for the rights of patients, and how frequently patient welfare is disregarded. The third section provides information that lies outside mainstream medical practice, including promising alternative therapies, useful supplements, and conventional treatments under development. This section will serve as a valuable addition to the medical advice that most patients receive.

Perhaps the most important lesson I have to offer is that prevailing medical practice constrains access to treatments that have a good chance of providing significant clinical benefits. Some of these options come from alternative medicine, which is typically scorned by conventional physicians. Others come from cutting-edge treatments, which patients often do not learn about until several years into the treatments' development—years that many cancer patients do not have. It is thus essential to pursue information and treatment options beyond the normal protocols. Intelligent patients who educate themselves can do a great deal to improve their prognoses. There are, of course, no guarantees, but conventional medicine provides none, either.

Medicine is not an exact science. Almost all cancer treatments are probabilistic in their effects, helping some patients but not others while causing considerable impairment and debilitation. The implications of this probabilistic nature are not, I believe, fully appreciated by oncologists. Even when there is a consensus about which treatment is most successful for a given disease, the likelihood that the treatment will succeed for any given patient is often quite low. Thus, rather than adopt a one-size-fits-all approach, it is imperative to identify patient characteristics that will help us predict which patients will benefit from specific treatments.

Oncology also ignores the critical distinction between diseases for which effective treatments exist and those for which effective treatments are lacking. In the latter case, the practice of prescribing standard treatments that have a known record of failure is simply foolish. Yet, for many cancer patients, the standard treatments are all that are offered. In fact, the current medical system actively thwarts access to promising alternatives—those in the early stages of development as well as those developed in other countries—even when credible evidence indicates that they may increase the probability of survival.

As I will discuss in later chapters, such treatments are unavailable because the U.S. government, via the FDA, has adopted a policy that rigidly divides treatments into "proven" and "unproven" categories based on a certification process of questionable validity. When the standard "proven" treatments fail, terminally ill patients are denied access to promising alternatives because these treatments have not yet received FDA approval. With the lives of thousands of cancer patients at stake, this is a vital issue. At this time in medical history, when the genetic revolution is finally beginning to pay off, it is critical that the system for providing cancer treatment be reevaluated and fundamentally changed.

Round-Trip to Hades

SECTION ONE

Forty percent of people will be diagnosed with cancer at some point in their lives. Cancer is a serious concern, especially for those who have a family history. In my own case, my biggest fear was leukemia, because I had two uncles and an aunt die of the disease. When I was in my thirties, I was convinced I had developed leukemia after a period of feeling really tired, then awakening one morning with greatly enlarged lymph nodes in my armpit. It turned out that I had a local infection from a splinter, and that my tiredness was the result of a persistent throat infection. From this I learned that being overly concerned about one's health can cause needless worry and anxiety.

After that, I rarely worried about becoming a cancer victim. My lifestyle was generally healthy: I religiously exercised every day, controlled my weight, and ate the right foods, although I will admit to an excessive fondness for good wine. (We now know that wine, too, is part of a healthy lifestyle, because it reduces the risk of heart disease and stroke.) I assumed that the odds were very much in my favor, and that cancer would never be a problem for me. Also, I was emotionally insulated from the prospect of developing cancer, as none of my immediate family or close friends had died of the disease. This changed abruptly in 1994, when I learned that a good friend, Richard Herrnstein (the famous Harvard psychology professor and coauthor of *The Bell Curve* and *Crime and Human Nature,* among other works), had been diagnosed with terminal lung cancer and had only a few months to live. I had studied with Dick as a graduate student at Harvard in the late 1960s, and he was by far the biggest influence on my intellectual development. I regarded him as the perfect role model for someone going into the academic world, not just because of his brilliance, wide range of interests, and thorough-ness of scholarship, but because of his intellectual integrity in addressing difficult issues that he knew would generate opprobrious reactions from his colleagues. I enjoyed his humor and envied his dynamic personality. I maintained contact with him over the years after leaving graduate school, and I returned to Harvard on numerous occasions thereafter, including a semester-long sabbatical in 1991.

I was shocked and deeply grieved when I learned of his illness. I had seen him and his wife, Susan, just a few months earlier, and he seemed robust and healthy. Soon thereafter, he coughed up blood, went to his physician, and was told he had only one month to live. In fact, he lived for three months. For a human being with such vitality to be struck down so abruptly can only be described as truly awful. Never before had I seen just how cruel fate can be, and how little control we have over it.

In the months after *The Bell Curve* was published (Dick, unfortu-nately, never saw it in print), the book became a sensation, appearing as a cover story in all the major newsmagazines. As Dick expected, it was harshly criticized, and it was terribly unfair that he was not around to answer his critics. No one was better at providing forceful and convincing rebuttals, especially in situations highly charged with political prejudice.

In January 1995, I discussed Dick's tragic death with my four siblings and their spouses at our annual family gathering. This particular meeting was in Gatlinburg, Tennessee, which is more or less the geographical cen-ter of my family (though my wife and I live just north of San Diego in Del Mar, a beautiful little beach town far removed from the midwestern culture of Kentucky in which we had been reared). It was cold and snowy in Gatlinburg, and, as we faced a dearth of interesting activities, we spent most of our time indoors. During this time I told my family about Dick's death. We began to consider our own cancer risks, recalling events from our childhood on a small Kentucky farm, where we were exposed to the various pesticides that were developed during the 1950s. My father was a county agricultural agent, which meant that he worked for the extension service of the University of Kentucky. Because his job entailed dispensing advice to farmers, chemical companies frequently sent him samples of their products. Of course, his children were the ones who did the actual spraying and dusting, and all of us had stories of being drenched with DDT, breathing fumes from Agent Orange, and more. We realized that we had received substantial exposure to some of the major carcinogens of our time, and that we would be lucky if none of us suffered the consequences. Little did I know that, at the time of this conversation, a brain tumor was growing inside my head. In a few weeks I would begin to have symptoms that foreshadowed a terrible disease.

Diagnosis: Glioblastoma multiforme
"The Terminator"[1]

CHAPTER ONE

MY WIFE, DIANE, AND I ATTENDED A DINNER PARTY HOSTED BY A colleague from the psychology department at the University of California, San Diego (UCSD). As a prelude to the dinner, our companions challenged me to a test. We had held a number of wine-tasting parties over the years, and I had gained a reputation as the department's wine expert. So, I was to take a blind taste test of several different wines. I passed the test with flying colors, but in the course of the testing consumed a considerable amount of wine.

As we left the dinner party, I had difficulty locating where we had parked the car. It's not that I didn't remember where it was; instead, my entire spatial map seemed reversed 180 degrees. Diane, however, was quite certain where we had parked, even after I insisted that I was right and she was wrong. Then, on the way home, she became agitated because I was not staying in our lane. When I focused on the task, I was able to get us home safely, though not without some difficulty. The next morning, Diane asked me about the experience. Although I hadn't felt intoxicated, I decided that I had had too much to drink and vowed to behave better in the future.

A couple weeks later I had another strange experience. Going for a run on a cold, windy day, I fell while jumping over a stream. I did not think anything about it, but then something truly bizarre happened. I was running into a strong headwind, with my body at almost a 60-degree angle. After considerable effort I realized that I could not continue, so I decided to stop. But I could not. As much as I tried to make my legs quit moving, they just kept going. I began to panic. Then I realized that I didn't have to stop to get out of the wind; all I needed to do was turn. And so I turned, stopped, and walked back to my house without further incident. Later I decided that the fall had temporarily impaired the neurological control of my legs. When I began to have severe backaches soon after, I imagined that this, too, was due to the fall.

A variety of other symptoms appeared in the next two weeks. Diane became concerned that I was parking my car erratically, and that I was walking with one shoulder substantially lower than the other. I was increasingly tired and finding it difficult to get out of bed in the morning. When I did awake it was almost always with a bad headache, but I had become accustomed to these due to persistent sinus problems. I also noted that I was making more errors while working in my laboratory. (I am an experimental psychologist with a primary interest in the learning processes of animals.) None of these symptoms caused me serious alarm until I developed problems with coordination. While I could walk normally when I made the effort, I often noticed that I was dragging my feet, one of the classic signs of neurological dysfunction.

Initially I thought this was due to an injury I might have sustained from my fall, but after a couple of weeks, Diane insisted that I make an appointment with my internist. I myself was becoming concerned, suspecting that I might have multiple sclerosis. On Friday, March 24, I called my internist, who offered to see me that afternoon. He agreed that my symptoms were odd and gave me a series of simple neurological tests, none of which showed any problems. He then referred me to a neurologist, but the earliest appointment was in three weeks. My neurosurgeon later told me that I would have been dead in two.

Concerned that I would be waiting so long for an appointment, Diane called a friend of ours, Dr. Leon Thal, chairman of the UCSD Department of Neuroscience (recently rated one of the top neuroscience departments in the world). Leon agreed that my symptoms were strange and that multiple sclerosis was a possibility. If that were the case, he said, there was no rush in seeing a neurologist because nothing was likely to change in the next few weeks.

Looking back, it must have been difficult to diagnose my condition. I was still mentally functioning with no obvious deficits, and my motor symptoms were bilateral. (As it turned out, the tumor put pressure on the motor tract running through the internal capsule, a part of the brain situated directly below and between the cerebral hemispheres.) Also, damage to the right parietal cortex, where my tumor was located, frequently causes patients to deny that they have any deficits. In any event, neither of the physicians I consulted were alarmed by my condition, so I was prepared to wait for the appointment with my neurologist.

Over the weekend I was extremely tired and did not feel well. My back bothered me a great deal, so we purchased a waterbed. When I lay down to test it, I felt so tired that it took a considerable effort to get up again. On Monday I went to work and functioned perfectly well. On Tuesday I went swimming, but I felt disoriented, as if I were in a daze, and I finally quit because it was eerily uncomfortable.

On Wednesday night a poker game was scheduled at our house. This was a monthly event that I had initiated several years earlier, when I was chairman of the psychology department, as a means of facilitating social interaction among the faculty. When I was an assistant professor, interactions with the senior professors were defined more by intimidation than collegiality, and I resolved to change the atmosphere in the department. Indeed, poker games helped serve that function. Very little money was at stake, but pride in outperforming one's colleagues, especially for the younger faculty, was a powerful motivator to play one's best.

In this particular poker game, I had more than my usual amount of luck. Poker chips accumulated in front of me, but how I dealt with them provided the final piece of evidence for my diagnosis. On my right side, the poker chips were neatly stacked in piles. On my left, they were in one big pile, as if I didn't know they were there. Neglect of items in the left visual field is a defining symptom of lesions in the right parietal cortex, where my brain tumor had originated. Oblivious to this problem, I remained in great spirits because of my record winnings. I went to bed feeling better than I had in some time.

A Trip to the Emergency Room

The next morning I could barely drag myself out of bed. After driving into work, I immediately went to my laboratory and began my usual routine. The experiments I was conducting were controlled automatically, but I had to place the rats into the experimental chambers before starting the control equipment. After their daily session, I would return the rats to their cages. In the meantime, I went upstairs to check my mail and encountered a member of my poker group, Brett Clementz, whom I had hired a few years earlier. After the poker group, Brett and the other players had discussed my symptoms and decided to do an intervention. Brett insisted that I go with him to the emergency room at Thornton Hospital, which was affiliated with the university's medical school. Though I was reluctant, I could not really argue with him after he showed me how erratically I had parked my car in the parking lot.

Upon arrival at the emergency room, there was a short wait while the neurology resident on duty was located. When he arrived, he repeated several of the tests my internist had given me the previous week, but now deficits were evident. The neurologist ordered an immediate MRI. This was my first MRI, and it seemed interminable. Although the chamber had an eerie resemblance to a coffin, the claustrophobia experienced by many patients did not bother me. What did bother me was the anticipation that something was seriously wrong and that I was about to hear some very bad news.

An MRI provides a series of brain scans that film slices of the brain from top to bottom, side to side, and front to back. For this particular scan, all three series were presented twice, once before I received an injection of gadolinium and once after. Gadolinium is a contrast agent absorbed by tumor tissue but not by normal brain tissue. If a tumor is present, the gadolinium appears as bright white spots on the MRI; the brighter the spots, the more rapidly the tumor is growing. It also shows how much tumor is present.

When the MRI was finally over, I began to assemble my belongings when the technician, Patrick, told me that the doctors would want to see me right away. From this I inferred that he had seen something very serious while conducting the scan. When I returned to the emergency room, the resident neurologist was looking at the MRI on a monitor. He was obviously having difficulty gearing himself up to break the bad news, so instead he invited me to look at the scan with him. I was horrified. The entire right side of my brain was infested with a tumor (see pages 16 and 17). After taking a moment to recover my composure, I commented, "At least it is on the right side." I had seen how devastating left-hemisphere damage could be. The neurologist approved of my positive attitude, but it was clear that he thought I would soon be dead.

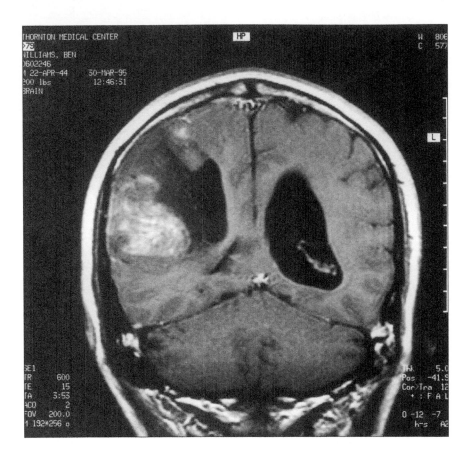

Figure 1

MRI slice taken midway between the front and back of my brain.

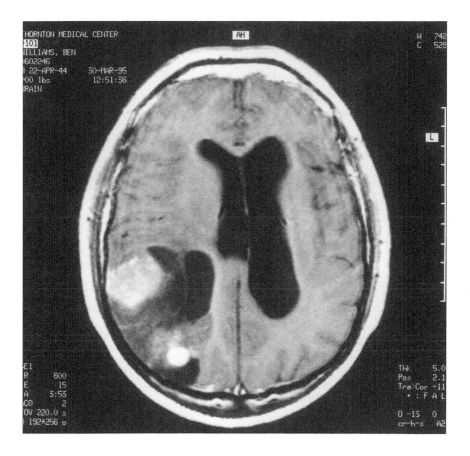

Figure 2

MRI slice taken midway between the top and bottom of my brain.
Similar amounts of tumor were evident on at least half
of the slices in both series.

Apparently, brain tumors as large and ugly as mine are a notable event. Soon half the neurology department had shown up to look at the scans. My neurosurgeon described the tumor as the size of a large orange; my neuro-oncologist later calculated its volume at 184 cubic centimeters.

Brett, who had been waiting in the emergency room, called Dr. Leon Thal. Leon gave instructions that I was to be immediately admitted to the hospital and that someone should contact my internist. My physicians insisted that I go to my hospital room as soon as it was available, but first I had to return to my lab to remove the animals from the experimental chambers and leave instructions with the animal caretaker. I met Diane back at the hospital, and we discussed getting a neurosurgeon. She called several of our physician friends for recommendations. They agreed that Dr. Lawrence Marshall, chairman of the UCSD neurosurgery department, was the best neurosurgeon in the San Diego area. He promised to meet with us later that afternoon. Diane, unfortunately, was not there when he arrived—she had returned home to get various items we needed for our hospital stay. Diane had requested that another bed be moved into my room so that she could stay with me, and the hospital readily agreed. In fact, we were treated extraordinarily well by the hospital staff. They went out of their way to assure Diane that I was a "very important person" who would be well cared for. They obviously were impressed that I had several physicians in the medical school looking after my welfare.

When Dr. Marshall arrived, he said that the tumor posed an immediate danger and I needed to have surgery the following afternoon. That night, March 30, was undoubtedly the worst of my life. I tossed and turned the entire night, not just because I was worried about the surgery and the possibility that I would be horribly impaired as a result, but because my anxiety had precipitated a severe attack of cardiac arrhythmia, for which I had a history. Even with a substantial dose of valium I could not sleep, and I spent the night pondering what was about to happen. At times I hoped that the arrhythmia might kill me, so I would not be subjected to the trauma that lay ahead. Having seen the extent to which the enormous tumor had invaded my brain, I expected that life as I knew it was over.

Surgery and Recovery

My surgery was scheduled for 2:00 P.M., but they moved me out of my hospital room at 11:00 A.M. because another patient needed the room. I waited in the prep area until my surgery. During this time, several friends and two of my graduate students stopped by to visit, wish me well, and inquire if they could do anything to help. It was a welcome distraction. I tried to make the best of the situation by cracking morbid jokes, which was my way of coping.

Finally, the nurse came in and asked if I wanted to be awake while being prepped for surgery. I told her no, that the sooner I was knocked out, the better. If my conscious experience was to be terminated, I wanted to get it over with. My anesthesiologist later told me they had considerable difficulty positioning the breathing tube down my trachea, a problem that might have been avoided if I had been awake to cooperate. The result was a severe throat irritation that persisted for weeks after the surgery, leaving me barely able to talk.

When I awakened in intensive care, the first thing I did was test whether all of my limbs still functioned. To my great relief, they did. I then realized that my greatest concern in the world was that I wanted a drink of water. Never had I been so thirsty. The nurse refused to give me water because she feared it would make me vomit and thus disable the various tubes connected to my body. I became increasingly insistent and was on the verge of pulling out the tubes and getting the water myself when she relented, bringing me a cup of crushed ice. I quickly finished it off and demanded another, and our battle of wills resumed. After several cups of ice she gave me grape juice, which was the worst liquid I could have received due to its viscous, grainy quality. Because of my previous obstinacy in demanding something to drink, I managed to resist vomiting.

I spent Friday night in intensive care and was moved to a new room in the morning. During this time, Diane asked Dr. Marshall how long I could be expected to live, assuming that it might be only a few months. To her relief, he replied that, while I had a malignant brain tumor that probably would kill me, it could be as long as three to four years before this actually occurred. His prognosis was based on a preliminary analysis of a sample of the tumor tissue, which indicated that I had an anaplastic astrocytoma, grade III.[2] Of course, we had no idea what that meant at the time, but Diane was relieved that I appeared to be in no immediate danger of dying. Over the next several hours, she reiterated how valuable these three to four years of life could be, although I was in no mood to share her enthusiasm.

Saturday, April 1, was my first full day back in a private room, and word began to spread that I was in the hospital. A number of people thought it was an April Fools' Day joke, then friends began to show up at my room. At one time it was packed to capacity, to the annoyance of the nurses who could barely get in to check the tubes connected to my body. Having an audience was great therapy, and I made numerous jokes about my encounter with the grim reaper. When I got up to go to the bathroom, I was oblivious to my bare butt protruding out the back of my hospital gown, which perhaps contributed to the humor of the day. One of my colleagues, Edmund Fantino, had been waging his own battle with prostrate cancer, and he encouraged me to go on a macrobiotic diet, which he credited for having kept him alive. As I had eaten at his house on several occasions, I joked that I would rather be dead.

The revelry continued until Dr. Marshall arrived and people were instructed to leave. Dr. Marshall had me perform simple motor function tests, the most important of which was to see how well I could walk. Though a little wobbly, I was able to walk relatively normally.

He then announced that I had recovered enough to leave the hospital. He would check on me the next morning before issuing the orders for my release.

That night, as my postsurgery emotional rebound began to wear off, I began to ponder my fate. The belief that I was in no immediate danger of dying provided some solace, but I realized that an ordeal lay ahead, even though I didn't know exactly what it would entail. I was distracted from my worries by a urinary tract infection caused by a catheter that had been inserted during surgery. The infection was far more painful than the metal stitches in my scalp, and even the narcotics I was given couldn't control the pain. It was only after the nurse offered me cranberry juice that the pain subsided. To this day, I can recommend cranberry juice as an effective treatment for urinary infections—not to mention its ability to counteract the pungent effects of eating asparagus.

Dr. Marshall returned the next morning, gave me more simple tests, and concluded that I could now go home. It had been less than three full days since I arrived in the emergency room. Brain surgery had become almost an outpatient procedure. The nursing staff brought me a wheelchair to take me to our car, though I could walk just fine, and Diane and I returned to our home. After we arrived, I slept on and off most of the day.

It was not until many months later that I realized how lucky I had been in avoiding surgical complications. A significant percentage of patients have an assortment of postsurgical problems, typically an infection or brain edema requiring steroids to reduce the swelling. I had neither of these, and I am grateful to Dr. Marshall for keeping me relatively intact.

A few days after my discharge, I returned to the hospital for a postsurgery MRI. Patrick, the technician, was surprised to see me walk in—he thought the next time he saw me I would be on a stretcher. After the MRI was completed, he mentioned that the medical staff who had examined the new brain scans were impressed with Dr. Marshall's resection.

The next morning, Diane and I met with Dr. Marshall to go over the MRI. He explained that he had tried to resect all of the visible tumor but did not go far beyond its boundaries. The tumor was so large that additional ablation would have caused serious problems with my vision. Glioma brain tumors have microscopic tendrils extending two to three centimeters beyond the discernible tumor boundaries, so it is extremely difficult to remove all of the tumor cells. Only the most aggressive neurosurgeons succeed in removing these invisible tendrils, often causing considerable impairment to the patient's ability to function. Because Dr. Marshall was more conservative in his surgical approach, my MRI showed that a significant amount of tumor remained (see pages 23 and 24). Dr. Marshall did not seem especially concerned about the residual tumor and commented that his colleague, Dr. David Barba, could treat it effectively using a type of radiation implant procedure known as brachytherapy. At the time I had no idea what he was talking about. I was preoccupied with the fact that considerable tumor remained after the surgery.

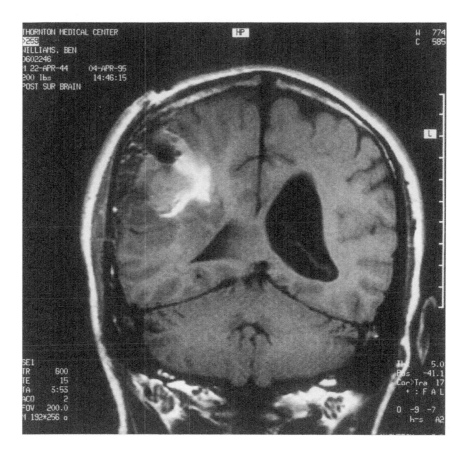

Figure 3

Postsurgery MRI slice taken midway between the front and back of my brain.

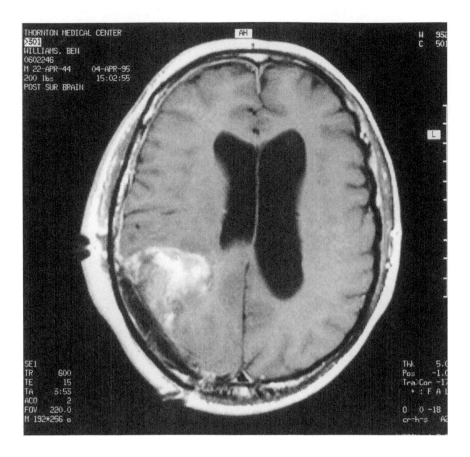

Figure 4

Postsurgery MRI slice taken midway between the top and bottom of my brain. Both slices show a considerable amount of tumor remaining after the surgery.

SURVIVING "TERMINAL" CANCER

A Bad Prognosis Gets Worse

A week later, we drove to University Hospital to meet with Dr. Marc Chamberlain, the neuro-oncologist to whom Dr. Marshall had referred us. Dr. Chamberlain was a member of the UCSD medical faculty. As he had also been recommended by our contacts at Harvard Medical School, we believed we were in good hands.

University Hospital in downtown San Diego was crowded, noisy, and totally lacking in aesthetic appeal. The majority of patients seemed very poor and totally overwhelmed by their situation. Needless to say, the depressing atmosphere did not add to our sense of well-being. In the examination room, Dr. Chamberlain gave me several cognitive and motor tests, which showed that I was relatively free of neurological deficits except for a small amount of weakness on my left side. We then waited while he left to retrieve the pathology report. Upon returning, he announced rather matter-of-factly that my brain tumor was a glioblastoma, the worst kind of brain tumor there is. He then cited some statistics: people with my diagnosis typically live about a year, but because I appeared to be functioning at a high level, I had a good chance of being among the minority of patients who lived eighteen months. His most positive piece of information was that I would not be in pain and would probably die in my sleep. His nurse, Patricia Kormanik, watched us intently, expecting, I assumed, an outburst of emotion. Perhaps that was the typical reaction to bad news.

Diane said she did not understand the discrepancy between what Dr. Chamberlain was telling us and what Dr. Marshall had said immediately after my surgery. Dr. Chamberlain replied that the discrepancy was unfortunate, but that glioblastoma was, indeed, my diagnosis. We then discussed treatment options, which included radiation and chemotherapy—the PCV combination. I had no idea what this entailed. He did not discuss the long-term effectiveness of the recommended treatment, though his forecast suggested that any benefits would be short-lived. He did not ask if I might want to pursue some other form of treatment. Instead, we were instructed to call during the week to make arrangements for radiation. Stunned, Diane and I left Dr. Chamberlain's office. I felt as if I had been kicked by a horse, which was perhaps appropriate given the horseshoe-sized surgical scar that occupied a good portion of my head.

The drive home was quiet but tense. Neither of us knew what to say; both of us were in shock from the new diagnosis and prognosis. We were in no position to think about how to proceed, so we rather blindly agreed to do what Dr. Chamberlain had recommended.

The next day, several members of my poker group visited, bringing me lunch. They asked about my diagnosis, and I was surprised that tears came to my eyes when I told them. All of us tried to be as matter-of-fact as possible, since it was clear that no purpose would be served by being morose. It would only get in the way of what I needed most—to develop the best strategy for dealing with my apparently fatal disease.

ENDNOTES

1. Holland, E. C. Glioblastoma multiforme: the terminator. *Proceedings of the National Academy of Sciences.* 2000;97(12):6242-6244.

2. There are several classifications for glioma brain tumors, but the most common distinguish between astrocytomas (sometimes referred to as grade II), anaplastic astrocytomas (grade III), and glioblastomas (grade IV). The life expectancies associated with the different grades vary by almost a factor of 10. Because of this wide variation, it is critical that the tumor grade be correctly diagnosed.

Searching for Treatment

CHAPTER TWO

THE NEXT WEEK I WENT TO WORK FOR THE FIRST TIME SINCE MY surgery. One of my colleagues, John Wixted, had already done some preliminary library work for me, gathering information about glioblastomas and their prognosis. I was looking for a glimmer of hope, but all the research suggested that a glioblastoma had no effective treatment and was uniformly fatal. I was impressed, however, with a paper[1] by Dr. Charles Wilson, who was the first to develop radiation and chemotherapy treatment regimens in the 1950s. Dr. Wilson spent considerable time discussing whether it was possible to survive a glioblastoma. Of the hundreds of patients treated at his medical center at the University of California, San Francisco (UCSF), a few glioblastoma patients had survived for five to ten years, but it was still possible that their brain cancer would recur and eventually kill them. There was also a question of whether these patients had been correctly diagnosed. In those early days of treatment, the diagnostic criteria were not clearly established, nor were the histological techniques necessary to assess the specific nature of the tumor.

When I finished reading Dr. Wilson's paper, I had mixed feelings. On the one hand, it suggested that at least some people survived for meaningful periods of time; on the other hand, there was little hope that the disease could be cured, and the odds that I might survive were bleak.

In the next day or so, Brett told me of his research on boron neutron capture therapy (BNCT), a treatment developed in Japan that involved bombarding the brain with neutrons from a nuclear accelerator. When Diane and I met with my radiation oncologist a few days later, he also mentioned this treatment, remarking that if he were going to participate in a clinical trial, he would choose this one. He also gave me a copy of a recent journal article describing the Japanese results.[2] The article noted that 15 to 25 percent of the patients treated with BNCT were long-term survivors, although some had severe dementia as a result of having BNCT after the standard radiation treatment.

Because everything I had learned up to that point offered no hope whatsoever, I was interested in BNCT. With Brett's help, I discovered that a clinical trial had just begun on Long Island at the Brookhaven National Physics Laboratory. When I called the person in charge, however, I learned that the procedure involved surgery: they would take a sample of tumor tissue to assess whether it had absorbed the boron molecules that would be targeted by the bombarding neutrons. I was not eager to have another surgery so soon. My interest declined further when I learned that I would be only the third person in the trial to receive the procedure. In the end, I decided not to pursue BNCT. This may have been a wise decision, since early results from clinical trials indicate that BNCT has no more success than the standard radiation treatment.[3]

SURVIVING "TERMINAL" CANCER

Monoclonal Antibodies

As I continued to ponder my treatment options, I received an unexpected call from a former graduate student, Dr. Jed Rose, who has become a world authority on nicotine effects and smoking behavior. (Among other things, Jed was coinventor of the nicotine skin patch.) Jed was perhaps the most interesting graduate student I have known in my twenty-five years as a professor at UCSD, and we had maintained both professional and social contact over the years. In fact, Jed had visited the week before my surgery. As we walked to a restaurant, I described to him my odd problem of dragging my feet. He was not disturbed by the news and later told me that I seemed entirely normal otherwise.

After learning of my surgery, Jed called to tell me that a colleague at Duke University was involved in a new treatment for brain tumors using monoclonal antibodies. With this therapy, antibodies carrying a small radiation load would target tenascin, a specific protein antigen found in glioma cells. The idea was to bring the radiation into direct contact with the tumor cell and kill it. Jed's collaborator agreed to send me a preliminary report on the first few patients to receive the therapy.

In the meantime I called Dr. Henry Friedman, the neuro-oncologist directing the project, but was told that he was on vacation at Disney World. To my great surprise, however, Dr. Friedman returned my call at about 11:00 P.M. that evening, which was 2:00 A.M. his time. He was extremely enthusiastic about the treatment and encouraged me to receive the procedure as soon as possible, which meant before the normal radiation therapy. I was wary, however, as I knew almost nothing about the procedure. I agreed to send him my MRI scans and histology slides so he could assess whether my tumor was suitable for the treatment.

A few days later I was notified that I was, indeed, eligible, but by then I had realized it was prudent to investigate other possibilities. Investigation on the Internet had turned up a few new leads, though most were in preliminary stages of development. I informed Dr.

Friedman that I wanted to wait until after the standard radiation treatment, which would last six to seven weeks. I would use this time to become better informed about my situation. He understood my reticence but explained that because his procedure required another surgery, I would have to wait two to three months after the radiation was completed, as surgery on recently radiated brain tissue is more likely to produce complications. Despite this problem, I still wanted to wait. We agreed that I would contact him when my radiation treatment was almost finished.

Radiation Therapy

My exploration of alternative treatments delayed the start of my radiation by two weeks, and I was anxious that my tumor might have grown considerably in the interim. I decided to receive radiation treatment at Scripps Memorial Hospital, which was located near my office, so I could avoid driving twenty miles to University Hospital every day. Scripps was not a participant in my HMO, and the treatment cost me several thousand dollars. This was my first experience with the world of HMOs.

I had been led to believe that radiation might be difficult to tolerate, as some people had nausea and headaches from swelling caused by the treatment. My only problem was that my surgical scar, which was in the middle of the radiation field, became so inflamed that it hurt to lay my head on a pillow. I tried vitamin E, aloe, and several other balms to alleviate the distress, but all were only partially effective. My only other complaint was having to show up at 9:00 A.M. every morning from Monday through Friday for the six to seven weeks of treatment. The sessions took only a few minutes each day. About halfway through the treatment my hair began to fall out, and by the end it was almost completely gone except for a few shocks in the front and back and some residual hair on the left side of my head. By the sixth week, I became much more sleepy and would nod off quickly unless something interesting was happening.

Throughout the treatment I did my best to maintain a serious exercise routine, and I even began jogging again during the last month. I also learned as much as I could about my diagnosis. I spent each day either working on PubMed, an online list of medical abstracts (and a godsend for any patient trying to become educated about a medical problem), or working in the UCSD medical school library, reading the complete articles that I had found in my PubMed research. It was an emotionally draining time. Virtually every paper I read began with a discussion of how truly awful my prognosis was. On one occasion, when I returned to my office after spending almost the entire day in the library, I lost my composure and wept harder than ever before in my life. Weeping had a remarkably cathartic effect, and I felt almost relaxed for hours afterward.

During this time I also subscribed to the BrainTmr interest group on the Internet.[4] While most of the messages were posted for emotional support, some provided periodic updates of individual cases. This gave me a sense of how the disease actually progressed, quite apart from the grim statistics I had read. A small minority discussed various treatments that different patients were undergoing. The case histories were often depressing, confirming my worst expectations. I learned about the demise of hundreds of people, some of whom I had become fond of though we had never actually met. Nothing is more depressing than to witness a valiant battle to stay alive, only to learn later that the person died in a dreadful manner. At the time, I felt this would be my fate as well.

Confronted with difficult treatment decisions, I decided that I had to keep my wits as keen as possible. I had been prescribed the anticonvulsant Dilantin immediately after surgery, since epileptic seizures are common with any sort of brain injury. The medication left me feeling fuzzy in my thought processes, and after about a week I developed a rash on various parts of my body. Dr. Chamberlain switched me to another anticonvulsant, Tegretol, but this made me feel even fuzzier than before.

I called Dr. Chamberlain to ask what might happen if I stopped taking the anticonvulsants. I was concerned with a phenomenon in the neuroscience literature known as "kindling," where the occurrence of one seizure makes subsequent seizures more likely and more difficult to control. Dr. Chamberlain told me that kindling had never been demonstrated in humans, but seizures could be quite serious if they did occur; therefore, he recommended that I continue the anticonvulsant medication. I decided that, as I had never had a seizure prior to surgery, it was worth the gamble. I quit taking my anticonvulsant medication, without incident. A few weeks later, I found a scientific study that corroborated the wisdom of that decision.[5] It showed that patients who had no history of seizures prior to surgery were no more likely to have seizures after surgery if anticonvulsants were not prescribed.

At this point I realized that medical practice was standardized for all patients, with little regard for the tremendous variability that occurs among individuals. While a given medical treatment might be beneficial for some patients, that same treatment can be counterproductive for others. For medical practice to improve, it is essential to consider individual patient characteristics when determining treatment.

Narrowing the Options

Midway through the radiation treatment, Diane and I had our second meeting with Dr. Chamberlain. By this time I had become informed about possible treatments, and I brought several pages of questions. Throughout the meeting, Dr. Chamberlain patiently answered my many questions, but commented toward the end that he felt he was being given an academic examination.

First we discussed the work of Dr. Burzynski of Houston, who had gained a substantial following among participants in my BrainTmr group.

SURVIVING "TERMINAL" CANCER

The medical community considers him a fraud and an opportunist, in part because his antineoplaston treatment costs many thousands of dollars. The FDA was in the process of taking legal action against him, which led to two different criminal trials; he was acquitted in both. Dr. Chamberlain shared the medical community's disdain for Dr. Burzynski and appeared alarmed that I was even considering the possibility.

The second issue I raised concerned a treatment involving Poly-ICLC, supposedly a broad-spectrum booster of the immune system. Dr. Salazar of Walter Reed Hospital in Washington, D.C., had reported positive results after using Poly-ICLC in patients with anaplastic astrocytomas (grade-III gliomas): all but one of his patients were alive after five years. His success rate with glioblastoma (grade-IV glioma) patients was not nearly as good, but still better than anything else I had read. When I described the results cited in the abstract, Dr. Chamberlain replied that such results were unrealistically positive and that there must be something wrong with Dr. Salazar's study. I accepted his assessment. A year later, the study was published in *Neurosurgery,* the most prestigious medical journal related to brain tumor treatment.[6]

The third issue I raised evoked a more positive reaction. I had been reading about the use of tamoxifen in brain tumor treatment by a Dr. William Couldwell of the University of Southern California. Tamoxifen is well known for its role in treating breast cancer. Dr. Couldwell had shown that, at very high dosages, it inhibited protein kinase C, an enzymatic process essential to the rapid growth of gliomas. After giving tamoxifen to glioma patients with recurrent tumors, Dr. Couldwell reported that about 40 percent had their tumors shrink or stabilize.[7] When I asked Dr. Chamberlain for his opinion about this new treatment, he enthusiastically replied that he was conducting his own clinical trial with tamoxifen.

At the end of our meeting, I brought up the possibility of Dr. Friedman's new treatment involving monoclonal antibodies. Although Dr. Chamberlain knew and respected Dr. Friedman, he did not think the treatment would work. He instead recommended brachytherapy, a procedure that Dr. Marshall had also recommended. With brachytherapy, radioactive iodine seeds are implanted in the tumor cavity and then removed after four to five days, providing a localized boost to the standard external beam radiation.

I spent the next two weeks doing intensive research on tamoxifen and brachytherapy. For tamoxifen there was only one paper, written by Dr. Couldwell, but there was extensive literature for brachytherapy. According to those studies, brachytherapy seemed to add about a year to survival time; however, the procedure was known to cause brain damage, and surgery was often necessary to remove the dead tissue. While it was comforting to know of a procedure that could keep the grim reaper at bay—at least for a little while—I was unwilling to inflict more brain damage on myself unless I were truly desperate.

Tamoxifen seemed the more attractive choice, as it caused relatively mild side effects. I called Dr. Couldwell for more information. Extremely gracious, he informed me that Dr. Robert Selker of the University of Pittsburgh was using a combination of tamoxifen and standard chemotherapy to treat glioblastomas. I contacted Dr. Selker's office and talked extensively with his nurse assistant to learn of any problems they had found with the combination. Based on these two sources of information, I decided that the risk in taking tamoxifen was minimal compared to the potential benefit it might provide. My enthusiasm grew after reading laboratory studies in which tamoxifen increased the effectiveness of both radiation and chemotherapy.[8,9]

Unexpected Resistance

I decided to begin taking tamoxifen along with the standard radiation and chemotherapy treatment recommended by Dr. Chamberlain. About three weeks before completing my radiation, I called Dr. Chamberlain and asked for a prescription. To my surprise, he refused to write it. Combining tamoxifen with the other treatments might be harmful, he said. I replied that it was foolish not to take a chance, given that the standard treatment would probably be ineffective, but he became increasingly insistent that I follow his advice. When I told him that I would get the tamoxifen with or without his cooperation, he replied that if I were going to develop my own treatment, he could not continue as my physician.

At this point I became testy, and it took a special effort to be polite. After all, it was my life on the line, and it would have been foolish not to use every treatment I could find that seemed promising. In retrospect, I believe Dr. Chamberlain felt it presumptuous of me to think that a few weeks of intensive research on my part could produce a better treatment than his many years of education and clinical experience. Perhaps it was presumptuous, but I had been dealing with intellectual issues all my life, and this was the biggest intellectual challenge that I had ever faced. I was entirely willing to consider all of his recommendations, but the bottom line was that his treatment was unlikely to extend my life by more than a few months. It made no sense to forego promising alternatives. Astonished and disappointed by Dr. Chamberlain's reaction, I told him that I would find someone to replace him as my physician.

Immediately after this conversation, I began calling the various physicians I knew for advice. I soon realized, to my surprise, that Marc Chamberlain was the only neuro-oncologist in the San Diego area. I then called my neurosurgeon, Dr. Marshall. Dr. Marshall had been at UCSD School of Medicine for many years. At one time he had handled the surgery and subsequent treatment for all their brain tumor patients. He had also been responsible for bringing Marc Chamberlain to UCSD and was clearly the authoritative figure among the small group of physicians who treated brain tumor patients. Dr. Marshall was sympathetic to my situation, and he offered to arrange a meeting with Dr. Chamberlain, himself, my wife, and me to iron out our differences.

I feared that Dr. Chamberlain would think I had gone over his head to complain to someone who was functionally his boss, which in fact I had, although that was not my intention. But as soon as the meeting began, it became clear that Drs. Chamberlain and Marshall had already discussed my situation. They had agreed that I could have more latitude in planning my treatment than was usually permitted. Perhaps this was in deference to my status as a fellow academic (with some important connections, including the chancellor of the university) and successful scientist in my own discipline of experimental psychology.

Dr. Chamberlain agreed to prescribe the tamoxifen, but only after I had finished my radiation treatment. The remainder of the meeting served no real purpose, although Dr. Marshall entertained us with stories about crazy things his patients had done, including one who died of liver toxicity after drinking large quantities of carrot juice.

Between our meeting and my next appointment with Dr. Chamberlain, I contacted Dr. Friedman to reiterate my interest in his monoclonal antibody treatment. He reminded me that his protocol required me to wait three months after completing radiation, and suggested that I might want to have a round of chemotherapy in the interim; however, to be sure that my blood counts recovered prior to surgery, I would need to wait six weeks after chemotherapy before receiving the monoclonal antibody procedure. This meant that I needed to have the chemotherapy sooner rather than later. Dr. Friedman also offered to set me up with an oncologist at another hospital if my relationship with Dr. Chamberlain again became a problem.

Brachytherapy

In the meantime, Diane and I anxiously awaited the results of my postradiation MRI. I had no idea what to expect, because my research indicated that any outcome was possible. Some tumors continue to grow throughout radiation treatment, and these patients typically die

SURVIVING "TERMINAL" CANCER

within a few months. Other tumors stop growing for two to seven months. About 25 percent of tumors shrink, but only a very small number disappear from their MRI due to radiation alone. I learned that a patient's response to radiation is a potent predictor of disease progression, and patients whose tumors shrink are more likely to have longer survival times.[10]

The results of my MRI were disappointing. While the tumor had not grown during radiation, it had not shrunk, either. I would not have much time before growth resumed, so it was imperative to proceed to another form of treatment. Dr. Chamberlain recommended that I immediately begin brachytherapy. He believed that the residual tumor was close to my corpus callosum, the fiber bundle that connects the two hemispheres of the brain, and that I was in jeopardy of having my tumor spread to the other hemisphere. If this happened, there would be little more that he or anyone else could do for me. This certainly worried me, but I needed time to consider my options. I doubted that I was in immediate danger, as my research indicated that I probably would have two to three months before the tumor resumed growing. By then, I explained, I hoped to begin Dr. Friedman's monoclonal antibody treatment.

At this point, Dr. Chamberlain became visibly angry. I tried to placate him, noting that brachytherapy and monoclonal antibody treatment were not mutually exclusive. Dr. Friedman had told me that brachytherapy was still a possibility, even if his treatment were ineffective. Because the chances that anything would work were low, it seemed only reasonable to take as many swings at the demon tumor as I could get. Our meeting ended with Dr. Chamberlain agreeing to administer a round of chemotherapy, as Dr. Friedman had suggested, while I continued to ponder my next course of action.

I contacted Dr. Marshall to see if another surgery might reduce the chance of my tumor spreading into vital areas. By now I was starting to appreciate the importance of the configuration of my tumor. It had begun near the surface of the parietal cortex, then spread back toward my visual cortex and downward to just a few centimeters above my midbrain. Dr. Marshall said that the residual tumor growing into my visual cortex could probably be removed, though at the risk of impairing my visual field. But he was adamant that the portion near my midbrain was inoperable because it was too near the internal capsule, a bundle of nerves that included the motor fibers. Surgery near that area could leave me paralyzed. Needless to say, I took him seriously. Additional surgery was not a realistic option.

Dr. Marshall did not think the tumor was so close to my corpus callosum that it would spread across it in the near future. He recommended that I consult with Dr. David Barba to get information about brachytherapy. In fact, I already knew a great deal about the procedure, which consisted of a mini-craniotomy to allow the insertion of catheters into the tumor site. The catheters were filled with radioactive iodine seeds, which were then removed after four or five days; this was followed by a convalescence of several days in the hospital to allow the residual radioactivity to dissipate.

I had reservations about undergoing brachytherapy. It would cause considerable brain damage, and it was not clear to me why the damage caused by radiation would be any less problematic than the damage caused by surgery. If brachytherapy resulted in necrotic tissue near the motor tract in my midbrain, then it posed the same risks as Dr. Marshall's surgery.

While pursuing my research, I discovered what appeared to be a better solution to my problem. A paper had just appeared in *Neurosurgery* describing a variant of brachytherapy that seemed at least as effective as the original procedure, and it caused considerably less necrotic tissue.[11] The variation used low-intensity radiation seeds, which were implanted just prior to the external-beam radiation treatment and left in the brain permanently. The procedure was reported by a group from Henry Ford Hospital and Wayne State Medical School, led by Dr. Laura Zamorano.

I contacted Dr. Zamorano to see if I would be eligible for her clinical trial, given that my external-beam radiation treatment was finished. She said that they had treated patients in my situation, but the treatment was more effective when the implants were in place during external-beam radiation.

It was clear that I needed more information about what would happen with the low-intensity brachytherapy alone. I learned that the procedure had been used in Europe with some success, but primarily for tumors with lower grades of malignancy. I also learned that the developers of the high-intensity brachytherapy treatment had tried the permanent, low-intensity implants in the early stages of their research, but they found them to be considerably less effective.

Next I contacted Dr. Mitchell Berger, then at the University of Washington and now the head of the Department of Neurosurgery at UCSF. One of the most eminent neurosurgeons in the country, Dr. Berger had been using the low-intensity implants in a clinical trial with patients who had recurrent tumors. We discussed the relative merits of the original brachytherapy procedure versus the low-intensity implants he was now using. His primary reason for switching to the permanent, low-intensity radiation seeds was that the necrotic tissue and the concomitant neurological symptoms caused by the temporary, high-intensity implants were no longer acceptable to him. When I asked how the new procedure compared in terms of survival time, he referred me to Dr. Alexander Spence, the neuro-oncologist with whom he collaborated on the clinical trial.

Dr. Spence explained that the median survival time in their study was sixty to seventy weeks—which compared favorably to the fifty weeks typical of the standard brachytherapy procedure—and that none of the patients had to have surgery to remove necrotic tissue. I became enthused that maybe low-intensity brachytherapy was a possibility after all. To learn the details of the study, I asked Dr. Spence to send me a draft of their results.[12] Unfortunately, the manuscript made clear that the low-intensity implants could not be directly compared with the high-intensity implants. Whereas the usual procedure used the implants as a substitute for surgery, Dr. Berger had surgically removed the residual tumor before the low-intensity iodine seeds were implanted. Thus, the results may have been due to the combination of surgery and implants, rather than to the implants alone. Interpretation of their results was further clouded by the fact that Dr. Berger had been more effective than is typically the case in removing the residual tumor. Postsurgery MRIs showed no evidence of enhancement for over 75 percent of the patients.

Because of the additional surgery required by Dr. Berger's procedure, and the fact that his protocol was approved only for patients with recurrent tumors, I realized that if I had brachytherapy, it would probably have to be the traditional, high-intensity procedure. Going that route still caused me great trepidation.

When Diane and I met with Dr. Barba, I wanted to know exactly how he would deal with the residual tumor near my motor tract. He thought he could do so with no problem, but I was still dubious. I asked how urgent it was for me to undergo the procedure. Would it be possible to wait the one to two months required for a round of chemotherapy, or might the tumor grow so large that it would no longer be treatable with brachytherapy? Dr. Barba agreed with Dr. Marshall: there appeared to be no immediate danger, and he saw no reason for me not to wait until after a round of chemotherapy before making my decision.

Impressed with Dr. Barba's low-key candor, I proceeded to get his opinion about other treatment possibilities. I had, in fact, attended a lecture by Dr. Barba a couple weeks earlier. He had described the results of a gene therapy study he had conducted with Dr. Edward Oldfield, one of the major innovators of brain tumor research. In this study, a tumor was implanted into a rodent's brain. Then, a modified herpes virus was infused into the brain, attacking only cells in the process of division, which meant that only the tumor cells were targeted. Later, a drug that kills the herpes virus, gancyclovir, was used to kill both the virus and the infected cells. The early research had been promising, but Dr. Barba was no longer enthusiastic about the infusion procedure because it did not cause the virus to make sufficient contact with all of the tumor cells. I found this information invaluable, because a human gene therapy trial had just begun, and I had been considering whether I should try to participate. Dr. Barba's assessment convinced me that this would not be a good idea. He also thought the same problem would occur with Dr. Friedman's monoclonal antibody treatment. In Dr. Barba's opinion, it was unlikely that the antibodies would contact a high percentage of the tumor cells because they would not diffuse very far through the neuropil from their site of infusion. I took this to mean that any attempt to use a localized application of a clinical agent was doomed to failure for the same reason. This message was discouraging, and our meeting ended with Dr. Barba apologizing that UCSD had so little to offer in terms of promising new treatments.

Tamoxifen

After meeting with Drs. Marshall and Barba, I was still in a quandary about which treatment to pursue. Perhaps as a way of evading the issue, I decided to proceed with the monoclonal antibody treatment, which would not begin for another couple of months. In the meantime, I would go ahead with a round of chemotherapy as advised by Dr. Friedman. I called Marc Chamberlain to inform him of my decision and to explain that Dr. Friedman had recommended a round of CCNU (also known as lomustine) instead of the PCV combination. Dr. Chamberlain instead suggested BCNU (also known as carmustine), because he believed as a single agent it was more effective. I accepted Dr. Chamberlain's advice and scheduled my first round of chemotherapy. Prior to the treatment I began taking tamoxifen, using a prescription provided by Dr. Chamberlain. I was concerned that the dosage he was using, 180 mg/day, was perhaps not sufficient, because both Dr. Couldwell and Dr. Selker were using somewhat larger dosages. I decided to supplement Dr. Chamberlain's prescription with additional tamoxifen purchased in Tijuana, Mexico, just across the border from San Diego. So, in late June, Diane and I traveled to Tijuana and began visiting various drugstores.

Shopping in Tijuana was unlike shopping in the United States. Prices varied enormously from store to store. When we finally made our way to the center of downtown, the cost was half of what we had been quoted near the border. Prices were subject to bargaining, even in the large drugstores, and I learned how to get the best price by purchasing several months' supply at once.

Back in the United States, I began taking the same dosage of tamoxifen that Dr. Selker had used in his clinical trial. I did not inform Dr. Chamberlain of the increased dosage. Given the difficulty I had in getting him to supply the prescription, I did not want to needlessly complicate our relationship.

Contemplating Death

Throughout these months, the realization that I was the victim of one of the deadliest forms of cancer never left my awareness. It was my first thought when I awoke and my last thought before I went to sleep. I would wake in the middle of the night thinking about my treatment choices. Did I have all the information I could get? What were the risks? Decision making was genuinely painful. I realized that I was essentially throwing dice with little control over whether I would live or die. Frequently I would give myself pep talks about living one day at a time and accepting my prognosis for what it was—the imminent end of my existence. I consoled myself with the idea that my early death was not necessarily such a bad thing. We all eventually die, and it is not clear that the latter years of most lives are really that enjoyable. When I was younger I had been impressed with Aldous Huxley's *Brave New World*, in which everyone was programmed to accept their death at age sixty without remorse. Death is inevitable, so perhaps it is better that it occurs early, before the ravages of old age inflict their miseries.

Of course, I did not want to die, and I could contemplate the end of my existence only with considerable discomfort. One can intellectually accept mortality as an inevitable fact of nature, but it is quite a different matter to lie awake at night anticipating the last moments of one's life and the disappearance of conscious awareness. As Woody Allen said, "I'm not afraid of dying, I just don't want to be there when it happens." But all of us will eventually face the grim reaper, with his scythe in hand, and the best we can do is accept this as part of the natural cycle of life.

When my friend Richard Herrnstein was dying from lung cancer, his friends were amazed at his tranquil acceptance of his fate. He said that he saw no more reason to mourn the inevitable end of existence than to mourn the fact that none of us existed prior to our births. I was not nearly so pacific. Like Dylan Thomas, I was not about to go quietly into that good night.

ENDNOTES

1. Wilson, C. B. Glioblastoma: the past, the present, and the future. *Clinical Neurosurgery.* 1992;38:32-48.

2. Hatanaka, H., and Nakagawa, Y. Clinical results of long-surviving brain tumor patients who underwent boron neutron capture therapy. *International Journal of Radiation Oncology, Biology, Physics.* 1994;28:1061-1066.

3. Coderre, J. A., et al. Boron neutron capture therapy for glioblastoma multiforme using p-boronophenylalanine and epithermal neutrons: trial design and early clinical results. *Journal of Neuro-Oncology.* 1997;33(1-2):141-152.

4. To subscribe to the BrainTmr listserv, send the message "Subscribe BrainTmr <full name>" to listserv@mitvma.edu.

5. Glantz, M. J., et al. A randomized, blinded, placebo-controlled trial of divalproex sodium prophylaxis in adults with newly diagnosed brain tumors. *Neurology.* 1996;46(4):985-1001.

6. Salazar, A. M., et al. Long-term treatment of malignant gliomas with intramuscularly administered polyinosinic-polycytidylic acid stabilized with polylysine and carboxymethylcellulose: an open pilot study. *Neurosurgery.* 1996;38(6):1096-1103.

7. Couldwell, W. T., et al. Clinical and radiographic response in a minority of patients with recurrent malignant gliomas treated with high-dose tamoxifen. *Neurosurgery.* 1993;32(3):485-489.

8. Zhang, W., et al. Enhancement of radiosensitivity by tamoxifen in C6 glioma cells. *Neurosurgery.* 1992;31(4):725-729.

9. Mastronardi, L., et al. Tamoxifen and carboplatin combinational treatment of high-grade gliomas: results of a clinical trial on newly diagnosed patients. *Journal of Neuro-Oncology.* 1998;38(1):59-68.

10. Barker, F. G., et al. Radiation response and survival time in patients with glioblastoma multiforme. *Journal of Neurosurgery.* 1996;84(3):442-448.

11. Fernandez, P. M., et al. Permanent iodine-125 implants in the up-front treatment of malignant gliomas. *Neurosurgery.* 1995;36:467-473.

12. Halligan, J. B., et al. Operation and permanent low activity 125I brachytherapy for recurrent high-grade astrocytomas. *International Journal of Radiation Oncology, Biology, Physics.* 1996;35(3):541-547.

Improving My Odds for Survival

CHAPTER THREE

IN OUR FIRST MEETING, DR. MARC CHAMBERLAIN HAD RECOMMENDED chemotherapy treatment without discussing the issues involved. It was only after my own research that I began to appreciate the conflicting views on chemotherapy within the neuro-oncology community. In short, it is not clear that adding chemotherapy to the standard radiation treatment provides any benefit for glioblastoma patients. The most widely held opinion is that it extends median survival time by two to three months, but a number of clinical trials have failed to support even this small benefit. As a result, increasing numbers of neuro-oncologists do not recommend chemotherapy because they believe that its meager benefits do not warrant the misery and debilitation it produces. It is important to recognize, however, that this controversy surrounds only the treatment of glioblastomas. For gliomas with lower grades of malignancy, such as anaplastic astrocytomas (grade-III gliomas), there is considerable evidence that chemotherapy provides a significant increase in survival time.[1]

Because my residual tumor remained undiminished by radiation, and because additional surgery seemed too risky, chemotherapy was my best bet for survival. While it is true that median survival time is only modestly extended by chemotherapy, a minority of glioblastoma patients (15 to 30 percent) do receive significant benefits. This is evident when we look at survival rates two years after diagnosis. Glioblastoma patients who receive only the standard radiation treatment have a two-year survival rate of 2 to 10 percent. Those who receive radiation plus chemotherapy have a two-year survival rate of 15 to 30 percent. The question was whether I might be among that lucky minority.

My research suggested that certain agents may increase the effectiveness of chemotherapy. Tumor cells defend themselves against chemotherapy by use of a pump-like mechanism that actively extrudes the chemotherapy agent from the cell. Because chemotherapy only kills dividing cells, this rapid extrusion decreases the likelihood that the agent will be present at the time of cell division. If the mechanism of extrusion could be blocked, it should increase the kill rate. Laboratory research with rodents supported this idea, so I spent several days investigating agents that had been shown to block the mechanism of extrusion.

Tamoxifen was one option, and my belief that it might increase the effectiveness of chemotherapy was one reason I had pushed so hard for it.[2] Calcium channel blockers, routinely used to treat hypertension,[3] were also a possibility; however, the dosages used to increase the effects of chemotherapy in animal experiments seemed too high to be used clinically, because calcium channel blockers greatly reduce blood pressure. Nevertheless, I felt that taking as high a dosage as was tolerable—in combination with tamoxifen—might be an effective strategy. I also wondered if I should incorporate another class of drugs that had shown a synergistic effect: the phenothiazines, which have been used to treat schizophrenia.[4] I chose not to pursue this after a UCSD colleague noted that the dosage I was contemplating would have a strong sedative effect.

I had scheduled my first chemotherapy treatment for July 5, 6, and 7. This provided enough time for the tamoxifen to accumulate in my blood. In the meantime, I contacted my internist to obtain a prescription for verapamil, the calcium channel blocker that has been most studied as a means of increasing the effectiveness of chemotherapy. I had mentioned my interest in the drug to Dr. Chamberlain, but he dismissed the possibility because there was no clinical evidence that it provided any benefit. My internist was more cooperative and provided the prescription with the proviso that I be careful to monitor my blood pressure.

Chemotherapy and the Blood-Brain Barrier

I had opted for BCNU as my chemotherapy treatment. BCNU, which became available in the 1950s, was the first chemotherapy agent used in the treatment of gliomas. The rationale for using BCNU is its ability to pass through the blood-brain barrier. Most chemotherapy agents do not.

The blood-brain barrier is part of the brain's defense system against potentially toxic material, but the barrier will not always protect tumor cells. Much of a tumor's blood-brain barrier is no longer intact, which is why the contrast agent used during an MRI provides diagnostic information. Because these cells absorb the contrast agent while normal brain cells do not, areas of enhancement on the MRI identify the presence of tumor cells; however, tumor cells in early development may not have a disrupted blood-brain barrier and thus may not be detectable on an MRI.

The same variability in absorption also applies to chemotherapy agents. Agents that are large molecules, such as heavy-metal platinum drugs, will contact tumor cells that have a disrupted blood-brain barrier, but not those with an intact barrier. As a result, chemotherapy might kill a large percentage of the tumor, but some tumor cells may remain. With a tumor's geometric growth rate, the small amount of residual tumor will soon expand into a larger tumor that presents significant clinical problems.

The role of the blood-brain barrier has important implications in the chemotherapy debate. Many different drugs have been used to treat gliomas, including *cis*-platinum, carboplatin, Taxol, and so forth. Several of these have shown a higher initial response rate than the traditional nitrosoureas (BCNU, CCNU, ACNU), but there is no evidence that they produce better survival rates. It is important, therefore, to know exactly what is meant when a clinical report indicates that a particular chemotherapy agent has a "significant clinical effect."

These considerations led me to accept Dr. Chamberlain's recommendation about using BCNU. Initially he had recommended a combination treatment known as PCV, which consists of procarbazine, CCNU, and vincristine. But the time required to complete the PCV regimen (approximately one month) conflicted with the requirement imposed by Dr. Friedman that I have at least six weeks between chemotherapy and his monoclonal antibody treatment. I agreed with Dr. Chamberlain that PCV was probably the better treatment, although the evidence supporting this was not very strong. Nevertheless, adhering to the requirements for the monoclonal antibody treatment seemed the more important consideration, so I proceeded with the BCNU.

Preparing for Chemotherapy

Everyone has heard horror stories about chemotherapy. Ten years ago, these stories were a fair indication of what patients could expect. Most patients experienced severe nausea and vomiting, followed by extreme fatigue and susceptibility to disease (due to reduced blood-cell counts). My neurosurgeon, Dr. Marshall, mentioned that some of his patients had found marijuana helpful in treating the nausea and vomiting, although he could not explicitly recommend that I use it.[5]

The conflict over the medical use of marijuana was a substantive issue for cancer patients until the early 1990s, when anti-emetic drugs such as Zofran and Kytril appeared on the market. These are remarkably effective in preventing nausea and vomiting, so there is no longer any excuse for patients to become immediately sick after receiving chemotherapy. Many still do, however. Some physicians do not prescribe the drugs because of the cost; others are ignorant of their availability. Fortunately for me, Dr. Chamberlain did prescribe Zofran, so my worst fears about chemotherapy were not fulfilled. In one year I received six rounds of chemotherapy, and I never became sick as an immediate result.

In preparation for my three-day bout with chemotherapy, I carefully read my *Physicians Desk Reference (PDR)*, which describes the possible side effects of all sorts of prescription drugs. Physicians often consult the *PDR* about drug pharmacology, and it is critical for patients to have this information as well. The *PDR* states that BCNU is supposed to be stored in glass bottles, not plastic bags typical for other intravenous drugs, and it should be shielded from light by a dark cover. Otherwise it rapidly loses its cytotoxicity. When I arrived to receive my treatment, however, the BCNU was in a plastic bag and totally unshielded from the light. When I noted the discrepancy to the nurses at the chemotherapy clinic, they consulted their own *PDR*s before returning the BCNU to the pharmacist next door to get it properly prepared. I did not view this as the fault of the nurses, who as a group were extraordinarily capable and conscientious. I realized, however, that patients need to be as educated as possible, and they must closely monitor the treatments they receive.

Our medical system is riddled with mistakes that appear innocuous but can, in fact, undermine treatment. Such mistakes can also be fatal. A recent government report revealed that almost 100,000 fatalities occur in hospital settings each year because of mistakes in drug usage.[6] Patients must become knowledgeable about the dosages and side effects of the treatments they will receive, and they need to be constantly vigilant to ensure that drugs are prescribed in the manner intended.

My BCNU treatment was a relatively benign procedure, with each session taking three to four hours. I occasionally needed to go to the bathroom, which required a complicated process of moving the entire metal stand to which my IV bag was attached. Otherwise I spent my time reading. Halfway through the procedure my arm began to ache, apparently a result of the alcohol solution in which the BCNU had been dissolved. The nurses turned on a heat lamp above my arm, and this was, indeed, effective. Later I learned that the ache reflected an irritation of the vein in which the IV was inserted. This led to blood clots that closed off the vein for future use, leaving a hard, thick cord that was painful to touch.

The matter-of-fact manner in which I endured my three-day stint of chemotherapy belied my emotional state during this time. I was alternately depressed and angry. To reduce the relentless pressure of the anxiety and uncertainty, Diane and I agreed that we needed a distraction. We found two lively kittens through an ad in the newspaper, the offspring from an unintended liaison between a Manx father and a Siamese mother. I spent substantial chunks of time playing with our kittens, yet even this did not totally alleviate my anxiety during the month between chemotherapy and my next MRI, which would indicate whether the chemotherapy had been effective. This was our most anxious time.

To cope with the uncertainty, I spent even more time researching the treatment of brain tumors. Even when the research was unproductive, I continued to believe, perhaps superstitiously, that I was getting the upper hand on my disease. Knowledge is power, and I was very good at acquiring knowledge. Fortunately, a few new leads developed. The most important presented itself almost by chance.

Combining Therapies with Low Toxicities

A member of my BrainTmr group on the Internet had contacted the neuro-oncologists at the M.D. Anderson Cancer Center in Houston, asking their opinion about tamoxifen, Poly-ICLC, and other new treatments that seemed less toxic than traditional chemotherapy. Dr. Victor Levin, head of the brain tumor center at M.D. Anderson and perhaps the leading neuro-oncologist in the country, replied that he was generally skeptical about the evidence supporting the efficacy of such agents. He then mentioned that his group had been using another relatively nontoxic agent, Accutane, which was normally prescribed for severe acne. The technical name for Accutane is 13-*cis*-retinoic acid (also known as isotretinoin), which is an acid form of vitamin A. Unlike most vitamin A, the acid form is not stored in the liver and therefore is less likely to cause the liver toxicity associated with excessive vitamin A intake. The M.D. Anderson clinical trial showed that Accutane, while not sufficiently effective as a frontline treatment, was active against glioblastomas and could be used as an adjunct to other treatments. Because Accutane was already FDA approved and thus easily obtainable, I resolved to add it to my treatment package.

I doubted that I could obtain a prescription for Accutane from Dr. Chamberlain, and it was certain that my insurance would not pay for it, especially given the high cost. It was only half as expensive in Tijuana, though, which meant yet another trip across the border. Before adding the drug to my treatment regimen, I contacted Dr. William Yung, Levin's collaborator at M.D. Anderson, to learn how the Accutane had been administered. I was told that the drug could not be taken continuously because the body quickly learns to flush it out. Their protocol was to use the drug for three consecutive weeks at a time, interspersed with one-week periods in which the drug was not taken. This was in important piece of information, because I did not want to be taking the drug while actively on chemotherapy. Like most forms of vitamin A, it probably had antioxidant properties, which many oncologists believed would counteract the effectiveness of chemotherapy. I could take the BCNU during the off-weeks, and thus avoid the possible problem. (In chapter 13, I discuss the controversial and complex issues surrounding the use of antioxidants during chemotherapy.)

My treatment regimen now consisted of tamoxifen on a continuous basis, verapamil in the one-week time periods surrounding BCNU, and Accutane in the periods between chemotherapy rounds. Only the tamoxifen presented any meaningful side effects: I began to have blood clots in my legs, and these had to be checked by ultrasound to determine their seriousness. Fortunately, the clots were all in peripheral blood vessels, presenting little threat that large clots might break away and lodge in my lungs. Through experimentation, I found that the clots could be controlled if I took two aspirin per day and long walks on the beach. The verapamil occasionally dropped my blood pressure to low levels, at which point I would lower the dosage, but in general I tolerated it quite well. Accutane had no side effects other than cracked lips and dry skin. All in all, the potential benefits of these drugs—especially given the real possibility that their effects would be cumulative—seemed to far outweigh their hazards.

We hoped that the combination of agents would improve my chances; nevertheless, Diane and I were extremely anxious when my next MRI arrived. We would not see the results until we had our appointment with Dr. Chamberlain, at which time we would examine them together.

For this particular appointment, Dr. Chamberlain's regular nurse assistant, Patricia Kormanik, was away on vacation, and Dr. Chamberlain himself was late. The nurse filling in for Patricia read us the radiologist's report. I was so anxious at this point that I missed the part about a shrinkage in a portion of the residual tumor; instead, I heard only that a large cyst had developed in the tumor cavity. I had no idea what this meant, and it added to my anxiety level.

When Dr. Chamberlain arrived, he was clearly miffed that the nurse had read us the report. He examined the MRI, then announced that there had been some meaningful reduction in the residual tumor. I was trying so hard to control my emotions that I had almost no reaction until he virtually yelled at me, "This is good news." Tears came to my eyes, and my enormous tension gradually changed into a sense of relief.

From that point on, my relationship with Marc Chamberlain lost its adversarial quality, and our interactions were friendly and positive. The fact that my tumor was receding rather than growing meant that he no longer pushed brachytherapy; it would not become an issue again unless the chemotherapy stopped having an effect. And, as long as chemotherapy was working, I did not want to undergo the mono-clonal antibody treatment, although I would not rule it out later if the need arose. So, we agreed to proceed to the next round of chemother-apy. Dr. Chamberlain urged me to begin immediately, even though the usual routine was to wait six weeks. It had only been four weeks since I completed the BCNU, but my blood counts were fine, and, as Dr. Chamberlain said, the tumor wasn't going to wait. This time I agreed to switch to the PCV regimen that he had originally recom-mended, as I no longer faced the time constraints imposed by the monoclonal antibody treatment.

On the way home from our appointment, Diane was almost giddy with excitement, but I was not nearly so sanguine. Typically, if chemotherapy works at all, it only shrinks the tumor for the first few rounds. Then the tumor usually stabilizes. My research had made clear that the only hope of survival was to eradicate all signs of tumor on the MRI. Small amounts of tumor that appeared stable for substantial peri-ods of time would eventually resume growth and quickly become fatal. I had learned this from an article published in the mid-1980s that pre-sented a compilation of cases at the University of California, San Francisco,[7] the leading brain tumor center in the country at that time. The analysis included only those patients who had an initial reduction in their tumor, and these were divided into those who had a "complete response" and those who had only a "partial response." Those with a partial response had a median survival time of seventy-two weeks, which was certainly an improvement over the typical median survival time of approximately fifty weeks. But patients who had a complete response to their treatment had a median survival time of almost four years. Half the patients died within a year after their first clean MRI, but the remainder were still alive several years later, presumably with a good chance of surviving indefinitely. Therefore, it was of paramount importance to continue my treatment until my own MRI showed no sign of tumor. I had a long way to go, but now I had a definite goal to work toward.

The positive MRI results reinforced my strategy of combining every agent I could find that showed meaningful evidence of treatment efficacy. In the next two weeks I added two more agents to my "treatment stew." The first was melatonin, the hormone naturally secreted by the pineal gland to control the diurnal cycle. Well known for its success in treating jet lag, it also has been ballyhooed by the health-food industry as a key to the fountain of youth. Its role in cancer treatment was pioneered by a group in Italy, where it almost doubled the survival time for patients with many different types of cancer, including glioblastoma. In 1995, the results of a well-controlled clinical trial[8] were reported in *Oncology,* one of the major cancer journals. I was pleased to discover the article, especially since melatonin is cheap, easy to obtain, and free of known side effects. Surprisingly, few American neuro-oncologists have incorporated melatonin into their treatment regimens. This is especially odd given that the presumed mechanism of melatonin's effect is a broad-spectrum boost to the immune system, which is sorely needed by patients undergoing chemotherapy.

The other new addition to my treatment package was polysaccharide krestin (PSK), a mushroom extract that Japanese physicians have used for ten to fifteen years in the treatment of cancer. It is believed that PSK provides a general boost to the immune system. It, too, has been shown nearly to double survival rates in well-controlled clinical trials involving several different kinds of cancer. But again, American physicians have ignored it almost completely. Unlike melatonin, PSK is expensive and difficult to obtain. The only source I could find in this country was a mail-order service run by a physician in Oregon. (See chapter 13 for a more extensive discussion of PSK, melatonin, and other drugs.)

Continuing Chemotherapy

With my tamoxifen, Accutane, verapamil, melatonin, and PSK, I proceeded to my next round of chemotherapy. I had chosen the PCV package, which was quite different from BCNU. It required three separate chemotherapy drugs, two of which were taken orally. On the first day of treatment, I took my dose of CCNU in the evening, several hours after loading up with Zofran. (CCNU is a first cousin of BCNU. Though not as effective as a single agent, it is less toxic with respect to pulmonary problems, which can be a serious side effect of BCNU.) One week later, I visited the chemotherapy clinic to receive an injection of vincristine. On that same day, I began my daily regimen of procarbazine, another early brain tumor drug that readily crosses the blood-brain barrier. Finally, after the two weeks of procarbazine, I received a second injection of vincristine.

This complicated treatment regimen continued throughout August 1995. The procarbazine component of the regimen prevented me from consuming alcoholic beverages. Given my history of having wine with dinner almost every night for twenty years, I certainly missed it, but my motivation to succeed with chemotherapy was far more powerful than my hedonism.

During the last week of August, we attended the wedding of one of my junior colleagues, John Wixted. The wedding was a lovely affair, but later at the reception I could not avoid feeling depressed. The contrast between the gaiety of the occasion and my own circumstances made me even more prone to contemplate my imminent demise. I could not relate to the happy mood, and I found myself thinking that it was just a matter of time before these moments of joyful human interaction would be at an end. I fully expected to be dead in a few months.

Later, while looking at the pictures taken at the wedding, I was astonished at how evident my depression had been. This was true for all the pictures taken during the first year after my diagnosis. However well we think we are coping, cancer exacts a heavy toll.

Shortly after the wedding I had another MRI. To my great relief, this one showed an enormous reduction in the residual tumor—I detected the change after only a glimpse. Now there was, indeed, hope that my treatment might succeed. I asked Marc Chamberlain if it were typical for people who had tumor reduction after their initial rounds of chemotherapy to attain a complete remission. It was not typical, he replied, but because my tumor had shrunk so dramatically, it was a real possibility. Diane and I left his office feeling exhilarated.

My blood counts after the second round of chemotherapy continued to be within the normal range, so Marc encouraged me to proceed immediately to my next round of PCV. Though I felt more relaxed about the routine, the procarbazine was becoming increasingly difficult to tolerate. I awoke each morning with a stomachache that was more or less continuous except just after eating. Forcing myself to take the pills in the evening became a real challenge. I began to drink milkshakes when taking the pills and at other times during the day, which seemed to alleviate my stomachaches for several hours. The vincristine was beginning to cause problems as well—my jaws ached and my toes became numb. I was relieved when the month-long ordeal was finally over.

During this time I continued my research, although I was finding less new information related to glioma treatments. I discovered a study conducted in India[9] and published in the American journal *Cancer Letters* in which an essential fatty acid, gamma-linolenic acid (GLA), was infused directly into the tumor cavity via catheter at the time of initial surgery. This resulted in a dramatic reduction in the amount of residual tumor in glioma patients. Even more impressive, there were no side effects from the GLA, and the benefits became evident within two weeks.

Impressed by the results, I assumed that the importance of this information would quickly be recognized by the neuro-oncology community in this country. I wondered, too, if it were possible to use GLA in my own treatment, so I began researching its effects on cancer in general. I discovered numerous studies that had been conducted in vitro (using cell cultures in the laboratory), but found none that had been done in vivo (using animal subjects). Unlike most countries, the United States requires that treatment efficacy be demonstrated in animal models before the drug can advance to human trials.

It was not clear to me why GLA had never progressed to the in vivo level of research and ultimately to the level of human trials in this country. At the time, I did not appreciate the rigidity of the requirements of our drug approval process. I naively believed that successful human clinical trials in India were grounds for taking GLA seriously in the United States. Except for the study in India, there was no meaningful follow-up on the laboratory research. I contacted both Dr. Barba and Dr. Marshall to see if I could interest them in the treatment, but failed. I then sent a letter to the American Brain Tumor Association, along with a thousand dollar check, asking them to encourage attention to the GLA treatment. I received a thank-you letter and a promise that they would look into the matter, but that was the last I heard from them. To this day, no one in the United States seems to appreciate that a promising new treatment has been entirely ignored.

Gamma-linolenic acid is found in several seed oils. Because it is nontoxic and available in most health-food stores, I decided to add it to my treatment package. The most common source of GLA is evening primrose oil, but borage seed oil has about twice the concentration.

I began taking ten capsules of borage seed oil daily, enough to obtain 2 g to 2.5 g/day of GLA . Of course, I was in the dark about the appropriate dosage, and I had no idea how much GLA made it from my GI tract to my brain. Nevertheless, there was no downside to taking it, except for the cost, so it seemed foolish not to include it.

Making Progress

My third postchemotherapy MRI occurred in late November 1995. Given the dramatic reduction on my previous MRI, I was hopeful that there would no longer be any residual tumor. This was overly optimistic, I knew, so I was only slightly disappointed when the results indicated that some tumor still remained, although it was substantially reduced. My tumor had two components, the largest of which was along the fissure separating my parietal and occipital cortex. Some of this still seemed apparent, although it wasn't clear whether it was tumor or scar tissue from the surgery. (Both pick up the contrast agent, so it is difficult to distinguish between them.) The second component was located much deeper, toward my midbrain. Dr. Marshall had said it was too close to my motor tract to be removed by surgery. To my great relief, this part of the tumor had almost disappeared. Marc Chamberlain commented that the remainder was in the process of breaking up. I did not know exactly what this meant, but I now felt optimistic that my tumor would soon be gone.

Because the side effects of PCV had begun to cause me trouble, I decided to switch back to BCNU. Perhaps this was foolhardy, given how well PCV had worked for me. I was curious, though, if the type of chemotherapy really made a difference, and I was not convinced that chemotherapy was the sole cause of my positive outcome. Moreover, I did not want to be burdened by the month-long regimen that PCV required, since we planned to visit Diane's family in Washington, D.C., over the Christmas holiday. I was not eager to make the trip—I knew my white-blood-cell count would be low at that point, and airplanes are notorious for transmitting infectious diseases—but Diane had not seen her family since my surgery. This was especially difficult for her because her mother had suffered a stroke eighteen months before my surgery and was bedridden. Also, Diane feared that this might be our last Christmas together, and she wanted me to see her family while I could. In any event, I finished my BCNU in the first week of December and we left for Washington, D.C., a week before Christmas. Unfortunately, I was not much of a guest; I spent two of the days in bed with a severe cold that I caught on the plane. After we returned, a blood test showed that my white-blood-cell count had plummeted to the point where I was classified as "severely neutropenic." This frequently results in severe complications that can be fatal; fortunately, I did not become sick again, and my blood count recovered over the next two weeks.

When the time for my next MRI arrived in mid-January, I eagerly anticipated that my treatments had eradicated the tumor. By now I had acquired a piece of equipment that enabled me to examine my MRI scans at home, rather than wait for our appointment with Dr. Chamberlain.

As I viewed the scans, I saw that the tumor appeared to be gone. There was some minor enhancement along the dura, the thick membrane surrounding the brain, but I assumed this was due to scar tissue from the surgery. Nevertheless, I was slightly anxious when we met with Marc Chamberlain the next day. He, too, was uncertain if the MRI showed tumor or scar tissue, but because the enhancement occurred in only one of the three MRI perspectives, he believed that my interpretation was correct. There was no enhancement in the regions of the brain where the tumor had been most evident, and I was convinced that it had, indeed, been eradicated. Diane and I were thrilled—the treatment finally seemed to have worked.

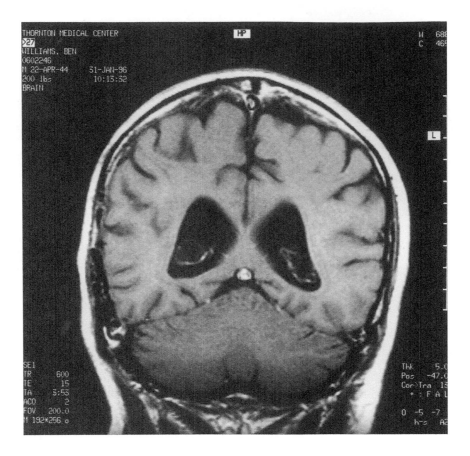

Figure 5

MRI slice corresponding to the slices shown in
Figures 1 and 3 on pages 16 and 23.

SURVIVING "TERMINAL" CANCER

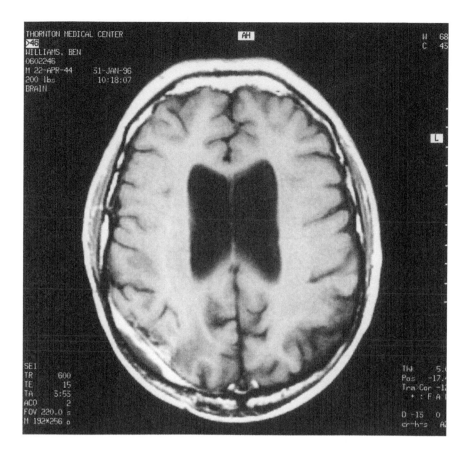

Figure 6

MRI slice corresponding to the slices shown in Figures 2 and 4 on pages 17 and 24. Although some minor enhancement is still evident, it appears to be along the dura, not in the cortex.

ENDNOTES

1. Levin, V. A., et al. Superiority of post-radiotherapy adjuvant chemotherapy with CCNU, procarbazine, and vincristine (PCV) over BCNU in anaplastic gliomas: NCOG 6061 final report. *International Journal of Radiation Oncology, Biology, Physics.* 1990;18(2):321-324.

2. Figueredo, A., et al. Addition of verapamil and tamoxifen to the initial chemotherapy of small cell lung cancer: a phase-I/II study. *Cancer.* 1990;65(9):1895-1902.

3. Bowles, A. P., et al. Use of verapamil to enhance the antiproliferative activity of BCNU in human glioma cells: an in vitro and in vivo study. *Journal of Neurosurgery.* 1990;73(2):248-253.

4. Aas, A. T., et al. Chlorpromazine in combination with nitrosourea inhibits experimental glioma growth. *British Journal of Neurosurgery.* 1994;8(2):187-192.

5. The fact that Dr. Marshall felt compelled to be so indirect in providing that information reflects a terrible fact about our legal system. In their efforts to restrict drug use, which have been remarkably ineffective, lawmakers produce unnecessary suffering due to their inability to make simple distinctions between medical and recreational use of the drug. Morphine is legal for medical purposes. Why should marijuana not also be legal, given its clear medical value? For this and other reasons, I have developed contempt for politicians who hope to gain political advantage by trumpeting simplistic platitudes about the evils of drugs.

6. Kohn, L. T., et al., eds. *To Err Is Human: Building a Safer Health System.* Washington, D.C.: National Academy Press; 1999.

7. Murovic, J., et al. Computerized tomography in the prognosis of malignant cerebral gliomas. *Journal of Neurosurgery.* 1986;65(6):799-806.

8. Lissoni, P., et al. Increased survival time in brain glioblastomas by a radioneuroendocrine strategy with radiotherapy plus melatonin compared to radiotherapy alone. *Oncology.* 1996;53:43-46.

9. Das, U. N., et al. Local application of gamma-linolenic acid in the treatment of human gliomas. *Cancer Letters.* 1994;94:147-155.

Salvaging a Life

Anyone faced with a life-threatening disease must contend with not only the perils of the illness, but its ramifications on every aspect of life. This is especially true for brain tumor patients. Brain damage can be devastating apart from the possibility that the tumor will kill you. The likelihood of physical and mental impairment—on top of worries about your loved ones, your employment future, your economic circumstances—adds yet more grief to an already overwhelming situation.

I resent being told that I am lucky. No one afflicted with a glioblastoma can be regarded as lucky under any circumstances. But there are degrees of bad luck, and certainly I have been more fortunate than most brain tumor patients. Despite having a tumor the size of a large orange, I have had remarkably little impairment. This was due, presumably, to the tumor's location in my right parietal lobe. But there have been deficits. It takes me longer to complete mentally difficult tasks, and I often lose my train of thought. My balance is impaired because the right parietal cortex controls one's sense of body location. As a result, I must be careful when walking down stairs, because I frequently have the sense that my feet aren't where they should be. I can no longer ski or ride a bicycle. And, since the beginning of chemotherapy, I have had greatly reduced physical stamina. But these are minor problems compared to what most brain tumor victims confront. Many deal with permanent disabilities resulting from brain damage, including paralysis, sensory impairment, and cognitive dysfunction. Moreover, the specter of a rapidly progressing disease often destroys any remaining quality of life before their tumor kills them.

I also have been fortunate in my personal and professional circumstances. Diane and I are both university professors and we have no children, so I had no need to worry about loved ones being cared for in the event of my death. We are financially secure, which meant I could pursue any treatment option that seemed promising without being constrained by cost. Because my job allows me to set much of my own schedule, I could devote a large fraction of time to finding an effective treatment and recuperating from my disease. The administrators at my university, from the chancellor down, were sympathetic to my situation, and they did not require me to teach unless I felt up to it. I suspect that when they made me this dispensation they didn't believe it would be needed for long, since glioblastoma patients aren't usually around for any length of time.

My scientific background allowed me to read medical journals and evaluate the clinical trials that determined the availability of treatments. I felt confident that my evaluations were at least as valid as the medical experts'. Although physicians have valuable clinical experience, few have the technical expertise of someone trained as a PhD in a scientific discipline.

I also have many friends who work in medical schools, which made it easier for me to find information about treatments that were in the early stages of development. Moreover, I had a great deal of help from younger colleagues who were more facile than I in using the Internet to obtain hard-to-get information. All of this gave me a tremendous advantage over most cancer patients, who have no choice but to accept without question what their oncologists tell them.

When I had my first clean MRI in January 1996, it was my first serious basis for hope that I might survive my disease. After that, I attempted to resume at least some of my normal activities, thinking they might distract me from my preoccupation with brain cancer. To an extent, it worked; nevertheless, teaching seminars was difficult, as my mind kept wandering to health issues. I often realized (usually too late) that I was not listening attentively to my students, and I frequently forgot what I had intended to say, sometimes in midstream. Yet, I could function—not at the level to which I was accustomed, but sufficiently enough to get by.

I continued to spend several afternoons each week in the medical school library, and I still participated in the BrainTmr group on the Internet. Both activities were depressing—the first because new and worthwhile information had become increasingly difficult to find; the second because more people I knew from the BrainTmr group were dying. I could have stopped both these activities at any time, which would have helped me refrain from my obsessive thinking and return to a more normal existence. But I knew that I was a long way from being out of jeopardy. Information, from whatever source, could be the deciding factor in my survival.

Although I resumed some of my activities, it was unrealistic to think that I could fully return to normal life as long as I was undergoing chemotherapy. Because my white-blood-cell count had plummeted after my fourth round of chemotherapy, I postponed the next round for a couple weeks in order to have a more complete recovery. Again I chose BCNU. It was easier to tolerate than PCV, and it was over more quickly. Unfortunately, a few weeks later I felt a burning sensation in my lungs, which indicated they were inflamed. Pulmonary symptoms are a potential problem for patients undergoing BCNU, although usually they develop only after extensive exposure to the drug. This was only my third round of BCNU, so I had hoped to avoid this problem. Now I was worried; inflammation can develop into pulmonary fibrosis, which can be progressive and ultimately fatal. To alleviate my concern, Patricia Kormanik arranged for a pulmonary test. It showed that I was still within normal limits, although the amount of oxygen in my blood had dropped significantly, perhaps because my hemoglobin level had been reduced by the chemotherapy. Nonetheless, the burning in my lungs persisted, especially when I engaged in any kind of physical activity. This persisted for several years, sometimes worsening from time to time, but finally abated in my sixth year after treatment.

The side effects of chemotherapy were not the only factor that kept me preoccupied with my medical status. As a cancer patient I was a frequent visitor at the outpatient clinics and the local health-food store. I had to have blood drawn on a regular basis, and I had to continually arrange for necessary drugs and supplements. Also, I was acutely aware of my upcoming MRI, which was scheduled in early spring. Then I would learn if my clean MRI in January had been a fluke or if I was, indeed, in remission. Needless to say, for the week before the MRI I obsessed about it constantly, trying to clarify in my mind exactly what I would do if my tumor recurred. After the procedure, I brought the MRI films home and Diane and I spent at least an hour going over every frame in detail. All were clear. I was in remission.

Our meeting with Marc Chamberlain a couple days later was anticlimactic. He agreed that the scans showed no indication of residual tumor and that I seemed to be in remission. Lest we were overly optimistic, however, he explained that the five-year survival rate for glioblastoma patients who receive a clean scan was only 25 percent. Most patients would have been discouraged by this information, which came from a recently published compilation of cases in Japan. But I had already read everything that pertained to long-term survival, including that particular study, and thought his evaluation excessively pessimistic. Moreover, no good purpose could result from deflating a patient's optimism at a time when everything was going so well.

In Marc's defense, the prevailing view among neuro-oncologists is that glioblastoma is incurable, and that it ultimately will recur. MRIs are an imperfect measure of the microscopic tumor cells that may remain after treatment, and any residual tumor can quickly expand into a larger tumor that grows with greater ferocity. This is a simple result of evolution. The residual tumor cells are those that survive treatment, so a growing population of such cells is less responsive to subsequent treatments than the original population. One or two clean MRIs do not mean that the tumor was eradicated, only that it was sufficiently reduced to be undetectable. If tumor cells remain, they soon will become evident on the MRI.

Only one in fifteen or twenty glioblastoma patients achieves a completely clean MRI. Their case histories seldom are reported except in terms of survival time. This crude measure fails to give a sense of the actual course of events for individual patients. Moreover, results among the few studies that have been published are inconsistent, perhaps because the patients who had positive outcomes received different treatments. I could find only one study that provided a relatively clear picture of what might happen to me from this point on. University of California, San Francisco, had compiled information on twenty-one high-grade glioma patients who had attained clean MRIs after chemotherapy, either BCNU or PCV.[1] Half these patients had a recurrence within a year after their first clean MRI; they died a few months later. But none of the remaining glioblastoma patients had recurrent tumors, at least within the period of follow-up. This meant that the next year was going to be critical in determining my likelihood of survival. After that, there would always be a possibility that my tumor would return. I would be living under a dark cloud for a long time, perhaps the rest of my life, but of immediate concern was whether I could make it through another year.

To buttress my chances of surviving, I was eager to get on with my sixth and final round of chemotherapy. My lungs still ached and burned despite the positive results of my pulmonary tests, so it seemed prudent to switch back to the PCV regimen. I knew that the procarbazine would again cause me stomach distress, but it would only be for two weeks. Then it would be over forever, I hoped. The vincristine also worried me, so Dr. Chamberlain cut the dosage in half. Even then I had neurological symptoms: my jaws ached, my toes became numb, and I had unpredictable sensations of prickling pain. Some of these symptoms continued for many months.

Life after Chemotherapy

I was relieved when the treatments finally ended. As I looked back on my year-long experience, I realized that I had been fighting a series of skirmishes not just with cancer, but with its various allies that attempted to undermine my health. Blood clots, weight gain, constipation, stomach distress, pulmonary distress, loss of libido, extremely low white-cell counts, anemia from low red-cell counts—each of these problems was manageable, but coping with them progressively eroded my resilience. It felt like one long sequence of low-intensity torture: no one part was intolerable, but collectively they sapped my mental and physical energy to the point where it was difficult to sustain any interest in normal human activities. I no longer enjoyed serious reading, and the only television I could tolerate were situation comedies. One year ago I had felt terrified of cancer, terrified of what lay ahead. Now its concomitant effects were progressively destroying my joie de vivre. But I did what I had to do. The question now was whether it was worth it.

My next MRI, in June 1996, confirmed that it had been. There was no sign of residual tumor. My third clean MRI in a row.

Now that chemotherapy was over, I vowed to spend the summer recovering my stamina. I had maintained a regular schedule of walking throughout my chemotherapy, but now I tried to resume running as well. Initially it was difficult—even a few hundred yards were beyond my ability—and improvement was slow. By the end of the summer I still could not run more than a mile or so. Before my surgery, I ran six miles every other day, and I occasionally ran in 10K and half-marathon road races. I had a long way to go before I regained my previous level of conditioning.

In the middle of the summer, Diane and I visited her family near Washington, D.C. The weather was typical of Washington in the summer—temperatures in the high 90s with humidity to match. The weather, on top of my general fatigue, curtailed my usual custom of visiting downtown Washington, and I spent most of the time in the air-conditioned house watching television. A few days later, Diane and I went on to a family reunion at a mountain resort in West Virginia, about a four-hour drive from Washington, D.C. This was the first real driving I had done since my surgery, and I was surprised at how enjoyable it was. The Roanoke Valley is an especially beautiful part of the country, and the mountains of West Virginia, with their switchback roads, reminded me of my experiences as a youth living in the easternmost portions of Kentucky, deep in the Appalachian Mountains. The weather was refreshingly cool, and even a solid day of rain was a welcome contrast to Washington, D.C.

I had not seen my family since the onset of my illness. After learning that my MRIs showed no sign of residual tumor, they interpreted this to mean that I was cured. They did not understand that my prognosis was still quite negative. Describing what likely lay ahead for me would serve no useful purpose, so I focused the discussion on the early events in my treatment. To my surprise, tears came to my eyes when I related my fears from the night before surgery. I had uncovered a deep wound that was so traumatic I could not recollect it without having many of the same feelings I had had at the time. People who have undergone intense trauma are probably never free of the emotions attached to it. They may try not to think about the experience, but when they do, it still packs a wallop. Perhaps that is what Freud meant by the concept of repression.

Shortly after we returned to California, we left again to go to Montreal, where I attended the International Congress of Psychology. This meeting is held once every four years. I was happy to go because a number of good friends from around the world were attending, and I had not seen many of them since the start of my illness. The conference was enjoyable, although at times I feared my presence was casting a pall over the meeting. My friends did not know how to relate to me; I appeared healthy enough, but they had been told I would likely die in the near future. People in general are uncomfortable when talking with cancer patients, because there is such a thin line between support and pity. I found that the best way to put people at ease was to talk about the situation as dispassionately as possible. A little humor went a long way, too.

When I was not attending meetings, Diane and I spent a great deal of time walking around the old city of Montreal. It felt more civilized than cities of comparable size in the United States—cleaner, less rowdy, no threat of danger lurking around every corner. I had one of the best meals in my life at the Beaver Club in the Queen Elizabeth Hotel. For the first time since my surgery, I began to feel like I had a reasonably normal life.

While speaking at the symposium, however, I was reminded of my limitations. My overheads and notes somehow managed to become disorganized, and I was forced to rely on my memory. It was the worst talk I had ever given, although no one seemed to notice.

My memory deficits became more evident after we returned from Montreal and I began teaching an undergraduate course on the history of psychology. In the past, my style of teaching had been discursive, covering various topics on my lecture outline and elaborating when necessary. I no longer could function in that manner. Unless I had my notes directly in front of me, I omitted large sections of the lecture and gave a jumbled presentation. I began to hate going to class, and my students' evaluations were the worst I had received in my teaching career.

Reevaluating My Priorities

Just after returning from Montreal, I had another MRI. To my relief, it, too, was free of any sign of tumor. I worried somewhat about a few bumps on the scans that looked a bit like warts, but Marc Chamberlain assured me that they were blood vessels, not residual tumor. Still, I wondered why they had not been detected on earlier scans.

Now that I had four consecutive clean MRIs, I assumed that my anxiety preceding them would gradually diminish. But even months later, when the number of clean MRIs had increased to double figures, I continued to worry. The stakes were too high. If the next MRI showed that the tumor had recurred, my life expectancy would be transformed from within the normal range to only a few months. How could I not be worried?

I continued to take an assortment of drugs and supplements while undergoing bimonthly checkups. Each new checkup was preceded by an enormous amount of anticipatory anxiety, but otherwise my life was relatively normal. My relationship with Marc Chamberlain became increasingly collegial: I kept him informed about my own research while he shared the latest developments presented at scientific conferences. I found Marc to be very knowledgeable, and I regretted that our relationship had begun on such rocky grounds. I also sensed that he had come to realize I might have something to offer him as well. To this day, however, I have no idea if the information I supplied was ever incorporated into his clinical practice.

For the remainder of the 1996–1997 academic year, I tried to resume my activities from the time before my illness. I found myself working in the laboratory virtually seven days a week and reviewing scientific manuscripts for professional journals. Prior to my surgery, I was on the editorial boards of all the major journals related to animal learn-ing and behavior, and I spent about one-quarter of my time as a consulting editor. But now I was rethinking my priorities. I was living under the dark cloud of a possibly recurring tumor. Did I really want to spend the rest of my life critiquing other people's scientific work?

Time spent at the laboratory was taking its toll, and I wondered if I wanted to continue. On the one hand, I had several graduate students who needed to do research in order to complete their PhD requirements. On the other hand, the cost of doing research had ballooned over the past fifteen years, primarily because of needless regulations resulting from the animal rights movement.[2] To continue my research, I would have to apply for a substantial grant from either the National Science Foundation or the National Institutes of Health, which had supported my research for the past twenty years. Grant applications take a great deal of work, and the time between submission and the point at which money becomes available is about nine months. There was a good chance that my tumor might recur before then and I would be in no shape to conduct the research once the funds were awarded. Why should I devote several weeks of work to projects that might never reach fruition?

In the end I decided to go forward with the grants, in part because I needed to maintain a positive outlook about my prognosis. Engaging in activities aimed toward the future was an act of faith that I would, indeed, have a future. More pragmatically, if I survived my disease, it would be easier to recover my life if I did not let my pattern of activity disintegrate further.

A Terrifying Moment

After each MRI, I would examine the brain scans at home on a slide viewer that I had borrowed from my laboratory. I did this because I always felt rushed when seeing the scans for the first time with Marc

Chamberlain. At home I could make my own detailed examination. If there were problems on the scan, I would have time to think more clearly, prepare my questions, and begin to plan my treatment. Of course, looking at the scans alone did exact a cost. Usually, Diane would not have come home from work yet, and the first few minutes setting up and viewing the scans were filled with intense anxiety. In many ways it was like playing Russian roulette. But as soon as I saw that there were no obvious problems, my anxiety would dissipate and I could examine the scans in detail.

A typical MRI consists of three separate runs of the machine. Each run records a series of pictures, slices of the brain that are a few millimeters in thickness. One set goes from front to back, the second from top to bottom, and the third from side to side. Each direction generates a page of individual frames, usually fifteen frames per page. It takes some practice to get a feel for how the individual slices add up to a coherent, three-dimensional picture, and I still am not very good at it. But if there are problems on the scans, they are easy to see. Prior to entering the magnetic resonance machine, the patient receives intravenous gadolinium, a contrast agent that is picked up by tumor cells but does not cross the blood-brain barrier of normal brain tissue. The gadolinium causes the tumor to show up as bright patches on the scans. Since my first clean MRI, I had no evidence of such contrast, but this was still the first thing I looked for.

During an appointment in early 1997, I noticed that the MRI consisted of four phases instead of the usual three. The fourth phase sounded very different from the others. (The main discomfort during an MRI is that the machine is extremely noisy.) When I asked Patrick, the MRI technician, about this, he replied that the radiologist was experimenting with a new MRI method called "flare imaging." He did not elaborate on its purpose, and I did not think anything more about it at the time.

When I arrived home to examine the scans, I placed the first page on my viewer. I was stunned. The page was filled with patches of bright contrast, mostly located in the area where my tumor had been but spread into other areas as well. It appeared that my tumor had returned with a vengeance, and, because it was no longer localized, it would not be treatable either with surgery or additional radiation. I would soon be dead.

After the initial shock, I walked around for a few minutes, trying to calm myself down. After all, I had expected this to happen eventually, and now I had to confront it. When I finally calmed down enough to return to my viewer, I looked at the next page of images. There was no sign of enhancement on this page, nor on the next page, nor the next. I then realized that there were four pages rather than three. Recalling the change in procedure during the MRI, I realized there was something odd about the fourth phase. Perhaps the new procedure was more sensitive, though I doubted this was true given that three of the pages showed no signs of enhancement whatsoever. I was enormously relieved, yet somewhat anxious to know just what the areas of enhancement meant. But most of all, I was angry.

We had our appointment with Marc Chamberlain a couple days later, and he, too, was surprised by the scans showing multiple areas of enhancement. When I related what Patrick had told me, he was irritated that the radiologist was conducting experiments on his patients without his permission. In fact, it was my permission that was needed, because any form of experimentation on human subjects requires their informed consent. This is a federal law that the university rigorously enforces. Because I was angry about being a guinea pig without giving my permission—and suffering extreme emotional distress as a result— I was tempted to make the radiologist pay for his transgression. It would have been easy to get him in serious trouble, because I was on friendly terms with the administrators at the university. But obviously no malice was involved, and the radiologist was unaware that I inspected the scans before he wrote his reports. I also suspected that Marc would make his own displeasure known, so I let the matter drop.

After this trauma, subsequent MRIs generated even more anticipatory anxiety. I was concerned about the enhancement evident on the "flare imaging" scan. Because it looked different than the enhancement typically produced by gadolinium, Marc felt that the MRI was probably picking up areas of damage to my white matter (myelinated nerve fibers) caused by the radiation.[3] When nerve fibers begin to lose their myelin due to injury, the process may continue even after the source of injury is removed. I was more than a little concerned that this might be happening inside my own head, especially given the frequency of my memory problems. But there was nothing I could do about it except wait and see.

Life-and-Death Decisions

Later that year, I asked Marc if I could have my MRIs every three months instead of two. He agreed, despite Diane's objections. She wanted to make sure that any recurrence was detected as early as possible, but Marc did not think it would make much difference clinically. I took this to mean that if I had a recurrence, it would kill me regardless of when it was detected. For my part, I simply wanted to reduce the frequency of anxiety surrounding the MRIs. I had finally reached a point where I was no longer constantly obsessing about my cancer, and the MRIs intruded a great deal on my peace of mind. Diane's opinion was the more rational: early detection can be important because there are treatments (such as radiosurgery) that are potentially effective when the tumor is still very small. These treatments are rarely curative, but they can buy time, perhaps as much as twelve to eighteen months. This extra time can be critical, given that promising new treatment possibilities are on the horizon.

Nevertheless, I opted to have my MRIs every three months. It was my best bet that my tumor would not recur. I had been convinced from the outset that the only chance for curing my cancer was to use systemic agents that would reach all of the tumor. A localized treatment, such as radiosurgery or brachytherapy, targets the residual tumor visible on an MRI, but the invisible tumor cells continue to grow. A systemic treatment, on the other hand, targets all of the tumor cells; thus, if the visible tumor is eradicated, the invisible tumor should die as well. So far, this analysis seemed to be correct. By the spring of 1997, I had had eight clean MRIs in a row. Surely any invisible tumor would have grown to the point of detectability by now. This reasoning was supported by my analysis of other glioblastoma patients: none of them had recurrences after one year of clean MRIs.

When I told Marc that I didn't think I would have a recurrence, he scoffed. Only later did I learn that he had never had a patient survive a glioblastoma, except for a couple people who had their tumors eradicated by brachytherapy. Of course, he had never had a patient who concocted his own treatment goulash. Though I was clearly in uncharted waters, I preferred my own assessment to his.

Believing that a recurrence was of low probability, I was eager to return to normal life. I had finished chemotherapy but continued to take high dosages of tamoxifen. After I learned how to use aspirin to reduce the likelihood of blood clots, tamoxifen caused me no real problems, with two exceptions: I had gained a considerable amount of weight, and the drug had completely eliminated my libido. Because of the side effects, I wanted to stop taking it as soon as possible. My dosage was ten times that prescribed for breast cancer, and even the lower dosage was documented to cause occasional but significant side effects, including weight gain, liver toxicity, and macular degeneration. I knew that the continued high dosage put me at risk, although exactly what that risk was could not be determined. Prudence dictated that I stop taking the drug as soon as possible.

The critical question was whether tamoxifen still was having an efficacious effect. By the spring of 1997, I had been taking it for almost two years. I knew that tamoxifen alone could inhibit tumor growth for substantial periods of time, and for a few patients it was responsible for eradicating their tumors. I took tamoxifen because I believed it would potentiate the effects of chemotherapy. Now that I was no longer receiving chemotherapy, it seemed plausible that tamoxifen was serving no useful function. On the other hand, I could not dismiss the possibility that my treatment success was due to tamoxifen alone. Perhaps it was preventing residual microscopic tumor cells from dividing. If this were the case, going off tamoxifen could be a fatal mistake.

Because of the high stakes, it was imperative that I get more information. I knew of only two people who had published the results of clinical trials using tamoxifen: Dr. William Couldwell, now at New York Medical College in Valhalla, New York, and Dr. Robert Selker of the University of Pittsburgh. I first called Dr. Couldwell to learn if any of his patients had obtained a clean MRI after taking tamoxifen. If so, did they continue to take the drug, and what was the result? In fact, he had only one patient who obtained a clean MRI while taking the drug. That patient had stopped tamoxifen after two years of treatment, and there had been no recurrence during the five years of follow-up observation. The other patients who had benefited from the drug continued to show evidence of residual tumor for sustained time periods.

Next I contacted Dr. Selker. He told me that three of his patients had obtained clean MRIs, and all of them had continued on tamoxifen after completing their BCNU treatment. All three patients had their tumors recur, with the longest remission being eighteen months.

Now I had information about four patients with treatment protocols similar to my own: three had continued on tamoxifen and had recurrences; one had stopped tamoxifen after two years and had no recurrence. Certainly this was meager evidence on which to base a life-or-death decision, but whatever its shortcomings, it did not support the idea that staying on tamoxifen was beneficial.

The old adage, "If it ain't broke, don't fix it," is certainly a gem of wisdom. But there was a cost in continuing to take tamoxifen. Even if

I did continue, I would face the same decision later that I was facing now. I did not want to take it for the rest of my life, and it was unclear at what point it would be reasonable to conclude that tamoxifen was no longer beneficial. There was no way to make an informed decision.

I resorted to using one of my colleagues, Hal Pashler, as a sounding board. Hal and I had discussed many of my treatment decisions, in part because he had an interest in medical issues due to his sister being a physician at the National Institutes of Health. Also, Hal had been an enormous help in my efforts to find information about new treatments. His counsel now was that I should continue the tamoxifen because it had not been that long since my first clean MRI. I finally agreed that caution was, indeed, wise, and I resolved to continue tamoxifen for another year. If I stopped tamoxifen and my tumor recurred, I simply could not deal with having made a fatal decision.

Getting to Know My HMO

Appointments with Marc Chamberlain were becoming increasingly routine. They were scheduled to last thirty minutes, but Marc's examination of my MRIs took only a few minutes, and Diane and I already had viewed them before we arrived. This left considerable time to discuss recent developments in cancer treatment.

In May 1997, Marc had returned from one of the two major cancer meetings where new research is presented. He reported great enthusiasm for several new treatments, most notably the new antiangiogenic drugs, which inhibit the growth of new blood vessels. I had been following the laboratory research on some of these, but I was unaware that they were now in clinical trials and the first results were being reported.

At that time, there were two major antiangiogenic drugs, TNP-470 and thalidomide. TNP-470 is a chemical cousin to fumagillin, a highly toxic antibiotic. Thalidomide is the notorious drug that caused severe birth defects in Europe in the 1950s and 1960s. Scientists now understand that the defects occurred because thalidomide prevented fetal blood vessels from developing properly. The growth of arms and legs from limb buds are especially dependent on the growth of new blood vessels.

Marc informed us that several other antiangiogenic drugs were under development, and that some had reached phase-III clinical trials. These new approaches marked a turning point in how cancer would be treated in the future. For the past fifty years, cancer treatment has been characterized as "slash, burn, and poison." Now that the biological revolution, begun in the 1950s, is paying off, scientists have a deeper understanding of the biochemical steps involved in cell division, allowing numerous targets for intervention when cells become malignant.

Although it was too early to know how effective these new treatments would be or when they would become available, Marc was uncharacteristically enthusiastic. Our discussion was energetic, and, toward the end of our appointment, he commented that our interactions had reached a level that he shared with his professional colleagues. I felt complimented.

This was our last meeting with Marc Chamberlain. At the end of the appointment he instructed me to contact Patricia Kormanik later in the summer to arrange for my next MRI. When I did, she informed me that Marc had abruptly left the medical school a couple months earlier, and that my case was being turned over to my neurosurgeon, Larry Marshall. I never knew why Marc left. He had had difficult relationships with some of the other neurologists in the neurosciences department, and, since he was no shrinking violet, it would not have surprised me if he had enemies.

I was unhappy about Marc's leaving, not only because I had come to genuinely enjoy our interactions, but also because the medical school had no plans to replace him with another neuro-oncologist. This was a direct result of San Diego's transition to an HMO-driven medical system. Even for a large community like San Diego, which has a population of over 2.5 million people, the number of brain tumor patients is relatively small. The patient base of a single HMO is rarely large enough to support a full-time brain tumor specialist. The obvious solution would be for HMOs to pool patient populations for diseases that have relatively low incidences. Instead, brain tumor patients are only authorized to receive treatment from physicians within their HMO. This means that treatment is determined either by an oncologist with no special knowledge of brain tumors, or by a neurologist with little background in oncology. The lucky patient may have an oncologist and a neurologist who cooperate as a team, but neither are likely to know much about brain tumors. Treatment recommendations may be several years out of date because most physicians spend little time following developments in specialties other than their own. All of this can result in an unacceptable level of professional expertise.

Brain tumor patients are well advised to go outside their HMOs to medical centers that provide neuro-oncology as a specialized treatment program. (Becoming a neuro-oncologist requires separate residencies in oncology, neurology, and neuro-oncology.) Unfortunately, many patients have neither the knowledge nor the financial resources to seek out a neuro-oncologist, a situation that is worsened if their primary care physician fails to provide meaningful guidance about what is in their best interests. These are frequent consequences of the HMO system—problems that have been ignored by our government.

Not having a bona fide neuro-oncologist was of no immediate concern to me. For the past year, Marc's primary functions were to prescribe my MRIs and tamoxifen, and to monitor my MRIs for signs of residual tumor. My neurosurgeon could serve the same functions, especially with respect to the MRIs. No one is better at interpreting an MRI than a neurosurgeon. Nevertheless, I was uncomfortable with the change. The disruption to my established routine only increased my anxiety.

When I called the Department of Neurosurgery to arrange for my next MRI and my appointment with Dr. Marshall, I found yet another reason to regret losing Marc Chamberlain. The neurosurgery

SURVIVING "TERMINAL" CANCER

staff primarily dealt with patients in acute need of surgery and perhaps a small amount of follow-up. They were not accustomed to patients who needed to be seen on a regular basis. Whereas Patricia Kormanik had handled all the details of my appointments over the past two years, I now had to get approval both for my appointment with Dr. Marshall and for the MRI. Dr. Marshall's assistant arranged for the MRI, but when I arrived for my appointment with Dr. Marshall, I discovered that it had not yet been authorized by my HMO. I waited for almost an hour before the hospital staff was able to sort it out. This was a minor glitch, but it added to my already heightened anxiety level.

I had learned from friends in the medical school that Larry Marshall was renowned for his forceful personality. While Diane and I had liked him from the beginning, I suspected that it might be difficult to reach the same level of rapport I had enjoyed with Marc Chamberlain. Surgeons are not known for their weak egos, and neuro-surgeons are the elite of the group.

Before our appointment with Dr. Marshall, we had what seemed an interminable wait while he inspected my MRI scans in his private office. When he returned, he was very friendly and announced that there were no problems. My MRI was "exceptionally clean," he said. This was all that I needed to feel comfortable with our new relationship.

ENDNOTES

1. See chapter 3, note 7.

2. This increase in cost is a direct result of the bureaucracy engendered by Congress's reaction to the animal rights movement. Even though every public survey has shown strong favor for scientific research involving animal subjects, the animal rights movement has found a receptive audience in Congress. The result has not been improved care for experimental subjects, who are treated essentially as they were before the myriad regulations were imposed. What has changed is the enormous amount of paperwork needed to show exactly what has happened to each subject, as well as new and entirely cosmetic requirements regarding the maintenance of animals. For example: cages must be washed at a specific temperature, and huge washers costing hundreds of thousands of dollars are now required for rat cages that could easily be washed down with a hose; laboratory-animal suppliers must be licensed and inspected, leading to dramatic cost increases (where once I could purchase pigeons for $1 each, they now cost $25); technicians taking care of mice, rats, and pigeons must undergo regular training in animal care policies, although their jobs are essentially janitorial in nature. Some of these requirements are so onerous that they would not be met by even the most conscientious pet owners.

In addition to the new regulations, an increasingly large number of bureaucrats have been designated to ensure that scientists abide by the new standards of care. In fact, it has always been in the scientists' self-interest to see that their animal subjects are well cared for, and humane standards of care were the norm long before the animal rights movement succeeded in doubling and tripling the cost of research. Ironically, animals that are protected by the government when inside the laboratory are considered vermin on the outside and are consequently the objects of government extermination programs. The methods used to kill these "vermin" are far more heinous than anything that could be dreamed up by scientists. When a rat consumes rat poison, it oozes blood from various body organs, a death much like that caused by the Ebola virus. Why should crossing the threshold of a scientific laboratory make such a huge difference in animal welfare policies? Inconsistencies in governmental regulations are not unusual, but, in the case of animal welfare legislation, the millions of dollars required to demonstrate compliance must come from funds that otherwise would advance scientific research, perhaps even lead to a cure for a cancer.

Stretching the available research funds has increased the time required for each scientific discovery. Cancer patients have a special interest in this issue, as virtually every cancer treatment that becomes available is developed using animal subjects. Now, when at last we are on the verge of major breakthroughs in treatment, any delay results in many thousands of deaths that would not have occurred otherwise.

3.   White matter corresponds to large myelinated nerve fibers that serve as the major channels of communication between the different areas of the brain. In comparison to the unmyelinated gray matter, which composes the majority of brain tissue, the conduction of the nervous impulse is much faster in myelinated nerves because the wave of electrical depolarization takes longer jumps along the cell membrane. Damage to the myelin membrane can result in the slowing of neural processing and cognitive function.

Toward a Rational Treatment Strategy

CHAPTER FIVE

AT THE BEGINNING OF TREATMENT, MY GOAL WAS TO DO EVERYTHING possible to attain a clean MRI. This seemed to be an essential first step to survival. But the transition from clean MRI to "cure" is fraught with hazard. The most generous estimates predict about a 50 percent chance of recurrence. Among glioblastoma patients, this is most likely to occur within one year after the first clean MRI. Paradoxically, lower-grade anaplastic astrocytomas (AA-3s) tend to recur much later. This presumably reflects the fact that glioblastomas have a faster growth rate (they are, perhaps, the fastest growing of any kind of malignancy), so any residual tumor not evident on a "clean" MRI will grow quickly. For AA-3s, the residual tumor might dawdle along for months before growing to the level of detection.

The fact that I was nineteen months past my first clean MRI seemed to put me beyond the period of maximum risk, and I was beginning to feel more confident about my treatment program. Upon further reflection, however, the grounds for such optimism seemed less certain. At the time of surgery my tumor had been classified as an AA-3; it was not until after a thorough histological examination that it was upgraded to a glioblastoma. This implied that my tumor was heterogeneous, including both AA-3 and glioblastoma components. I might be beyond the threat of the glioblastoma, but the AA-3 component still had a significant chance of recurring over the next several years. In the event of a recurrence, I needed a contingency plan.

Throughout my research, I tried to find as many agents as possible that were shown to have at least some efficacy. If you combine a half-dozen treatments, each of which seems to significantly help 20 to 40 percent of patients, then the laws of probability imply that their aggregate effect should be well above the 50 percent level. In time, however, I became convinced that the combined effect should be much higher.

HIV and Cancer

Consider the similarity between AIDS and cancer. The HIV virus and cancer cells are biological entities that mutate rapidly. Because mutations can develop resistance to treatment agents, treatments for these diseases often seem effective at first but may become less effective over time.

The major advance in AIDS treatment was the discovery that a combination of agents is more effective in overcoming this resistance than individual agents. When a mutated cell becomes resistant to a treatment agent, that resistance is transmitted to subsequent generations of cells. The result is a virulent cell population that is much less likely to respond to the treatment in the future. But when that same treatment is part of a treatment "cocktail" along with several other agents having different mechanisms of action, the other agents can prevent the cell from dividing, causing the mutation to "die on the vine." It seemed that the same concept could apply to cancer cells. Perhaps my outcome had been successful because I used a drug cocktail that included agents with different mechanisms of action, and this prevented my tumor from developing resistance to my treatments.

I was impressed by another detail related to AIDS treatment: the development of AZT. As an early approach to treating HIV, AZT showed great promise, but optimism quickly changed to disappointment as most patients developed resistance to the drug. When those patients were switched to drug cocktails, their outcomes were significantly worse than patients who had not had prior exposure to AZT. If the analogy between AIDS and cancer is valid, this implies that simultaneous drug combinations are best used as the initial approach to treatment, not after individual treatment agents are shown to fail. Yet, the typical approach to glioblastoma treatment is to prescribe the single "best" agent (which historically has been BCNU), then, after it fails, to prescribe another drug (such as procarbazine), and so on until the patient's vital resources are depleted. Such an approach will never exploit the synergistic effects of combined treatments, thus depriving patients of their best chance for survival.

There are at least two difficulties in using drug cocktails to treat brain tumors. First, other than radiation, treatments prescribed by neuro-oncologists are mainly limited to varieties of chemotherapy, each of which is highly toxic. Different types of chemotherapy have different toxicity profiles, which is the basis for the successful combination of chemotherapy agents to treat certain types of cancer (such as childhood leukemia). But drugs known to benefit brain tumor patients have similar toxicity profiles. Any positive effects of combining these drugs are offset by the cumulative toxicity, especially with respect to both white-cell and red-cell counts.

This problem seemed less imposing than it had when I began my treatment. After a few months of research, I had identified a half-dozen new treatments that showed some effect against gliomas without the cytotoxic effects of chemotherapy. Among these were tamoxifen, Accutane (13-*cis*-retinoic acid), gamma-linolenic acid, and melatonin, all of which I incorporated into my treatment package. (I also included PSK based on evidence that it improved patient outcome for various kinds of cancer, although it had not been studied with brain tumors, per se.) Combining chemotherapy with these other drugs may have created a manageable level of toxicity as well as a synergistic effect analogous to that of the AIDS cocktail.

The second difficulty in implementing a drug cocktail approach is understanding the interactions among treatment agents. When drugs are combined, there is always a risk of negative interactions. But when your neuro-oncologist tells you that your disease is incurable, this risk seems dim when compared to the hope of finding a life-saving treatment. Nevertheless, it is important to minimize that risk as much as possible.

For every drug I added to my treatment regimen, I read all of the available literature to understand how the drug worked and what kind of deleterious effects it might have. To my surprise, all of the agents I chose seemed to work by different mechanisms, and there was no reason to expect an adverse interaction. Tamoxifen inhibits tumor growth because it suppresses protein kinase C, an enzymatic process that propels the hyperactive cell division in gliomas. Tamoxifen also augments the effects of chemotherapy by slowing the extrusion of chemotherapy agents from cancer cells.[1] Accutane blocks the receptor for the epidermal growth factor signal, a second catalyst in glioma cell division,[2] and it activates various genes that cause cancer cells to differentiate into normal cells that do not wildly divide. Melatonin and PSK boost the immune system. Gamma-linolenic acid not only produces a lethal level of free radicals inside cancer cells, but also activates genes that produce cell differentiation.

Of course, my research was riddled with speculation. Mechanisms of action were not strongly established for any of these agents, and there was no hard evidence about possible interactions. Though my best calculations showed only a small possibility of potentially dangerous drug interactions, I was sailing in uncharted waters. I realized that my hypotheses were based on an empirically flimsy foundation. Perhaps the chemotherapy alone had eradicated my tumor, and the rest of my treatment was only window dressing. If so, I was in the same boat as other patients who had achieved clean MRIs: there was a good possibility that my tumor would recur. I continued to be on the lookout for new treatments that held the promise of being effective.

The Wave of the Future

At one of our last appointments with Marc Chamberlain, Marc had just returned from a meeting of the American Society of Clinical Oncology, one of two major national meetings of cancer researchers. I had read the proceedings of these meetings for several years—they provide the most up-to-date information about ongoing research, which typically does not appear in the professional journals until one to three years later. For a cancer patient with a lethal diagnosis, this time lag is, quite literally, an eternity. Even when a new treatment reaches the beginning stages of clinical investigation, a cancer patient is likely to die before it actually becomes available.

When Marc returned from the meeting, he was uncharacteristically excited about two new approaches to glioblastoma treatment: metalloproteinase inhibitors and antiangiogenic agents. These approaches were inspired by advances in biology that allowed scientists to better understand the complex processes involved in cell division and in how tumor cells invade adjacent normal tissue. Unlike chemotherapy, which kills any type of dividing cell, these new treatments target specific processes underlying the malignant growth unique to cancer cells. Tamoxifen and Accutane fall into this category of treatment, but the two new approaches discussed at the meeting were potentially more powerful in their therapeutic effects.

Myriad processes are involved in the proliferation of cancer cells. The more we understand these processes, the more we can identify opportunities for intervention. For example, in order for a tumor to grow, its cells must break down the matrix of adjacent normal cells, in essence digesting the cell matrix to make space for growth. Because metalloproteinase enzymes are involved in this breakdown, chemicals that inhibit this enzymatic process should be able to hold the cancer proliferation in check. For a tumor to grow larger than the size of a pinhead, it must recruit tiny blood vessels that provide a blood supply, a process known as angiogenesis. Antiangiogenic drugs inhibit the growth of new blood vessels, preventing access to the blood supply necessary to sustain tumor growth.[3] The logic is similar to a military strategy that concentrates on the enemy's supply lines rather than on a direct frontal assault.

Marc had learned that the first wave of metalloproteinase inhibitors were already being investigated in human clinical trials. He had been invited to participate in the final phase-III trial, in which one of these inhibitors, marimastat, would be randomly given to one group while a second group received only a placebo. Uncomfortable with the idea of a placebo control, Marc turned the offer down. Nevertheless, he was impressed with the enthusiasm of those involved with the project, and in their belief that this could be a major breakthrough.

When Marc told us that new treatments may be on the horizon, I felt enormous relief. Perhaps I could finally escape the dark cloud I had been living under. Maybe there was, indeed, going to be a cure for cancer, however unbelievable this had seemed three years ago.

I immediately began researching the new treatments that Marc had described. None of them had yet appeared in scientific journals, but there were abstracts available of research presented at scientific meetings. In addition, the small biotech companies that sponsored much of the research reported information about these agents on their Web sites. Phase-III results for marimastat, the metalloproteinase inhibitor, were scheduled for release in 1999. (Unfortunately, the trials would show that the treatment did not produce an improvement in survival time.)

I learned that TNP-470 and thalidomide, the antiangiogenic agents, were also in clinical trials. I tried to find information about TNP-470's clinical trials, but there were no published data. The company that owned the drug, Tap Pharmaceuticals, was unresponsive to my inquiries, which I took to be a bad omen about the drug's potential usefulness. I was already familiar with the other agent, thalidomide, which had caused severe birth defects in Europe in the 1950s and 1960s. Originally prescribed to combat morning sickness in pregnant women, thalidomide prevented fetal blood vessels from developing properly. Because the growth of limbs is especially dependent on the growth of new blood vessels, babies exposed to thalidomide were born with deformed arms and legs. The drug was quickly outlawed when the teratological effects were discovered, and it was never approved for clinical use in the United States. Now thalidomide was being resurrected as a cancer treatment for exactly the same reason it had caused birth defects: it prevented the formation of new blood vessels.

For me, the critical question was whether thalidomide would be effective in the event of a recurrence. It was the subject of three separate clinical trials conducted by EntreMed, a small biotech company in Bethesda, Maryland, near the National Cancer Institute. EntreMed had acquired the rights to the antiangiogenic drugs being developed by Dr. Judah Folkman at Harvard; in return, they agreed to provide financial support for all his research.[4]

The thalidomide trials, which involved Kaposi's sarcoma, metastatic prostate cancer, and glioblastoma, were used to test the idea of antiangiogenesis as a cancer treatment. Although the results, reported in the spring of 1997, were not spectacular,[5] all of the trials showed some degree of efficacy, validating antiangiogenesis as a potential treatment for cancer. Newer antiangiogenic drugs were in the pipeline, and these were expected to be much more potent.

I was primarily interested in the glioblastoma trial. Its principal investigator was Dr. Howard Fine at the Dana-Farber Cancer Institute in Boston. Dr. Fine and his collaborators reported that 40 to 50 percent of patients with recurrent glioblastoma had their tumors stop growing or shrink.[6] The stabilization periods were relatively short—no better or worse than available treatments for recurrent glioblastoma—but the thalidomide allowed patients to avoid the pitfalls of chemotherapy.

Shortly after Dr. Fine's clinical trial, I learned of a second trial being conducted by Drs. Michael Gruber and Jon Glass at New York University. Unlike Dr. Fine's trial, which used thalidomide as a single agent, the NYU trial combined thalidomide with carboplatin, one of the most widely used chemotherapy drugs. I read about this clinical trial in the Parade section of my Sunday newspaper, of all places. The report stated that the first three patients to receive this combination showed no sign of residual tumor after the treatment. This seemed too good to be true, so several members of my BrainTmr group contacted Dr. Gruber's clinic to verify it. Indeed, the report was an exaggeration; the more complete data indicated that 65 percent of the patients with recurrent glioblastoma had their tumors regress or stabilize, and the median survival time was ten months.[7] Not the wonder cure everyone had hoped for, but it seemed more promising than the conventional treatment for recurrent glioblastoma, which offered a survival time of three to four months.

Antiangiogenic drugs seemed to be the wave of the future. For now, though, I needed to plan on the basis of what was available today—not what might be available in one or two years. I now had the following information:

- Thalidomide alone helped 40 to 50 percent of glioblastoma patients.
- Thalidomide in combination with carboplatin seemed to produce an even better outcome.
- Tamoxifen alone significantly helped 30 to 40 percent of glioma patients.
- Tamoxifen in combination with carboplatin seemed more effective than tamoxifen alone.

SURVIVING "TERMINAL" CANCER

- Accutane (13-*cis*-retinoic acid) significantly helped 30 to 45 percent of glioblastoma patients, with positive effects often lasting more than a year.
- Melatonin alone doubled the survival time for glioblastoma patients relative to those who received only radiation.

In addition, I strongly suspected that gamma-linolenic acid and PSK, the mushroom extract from Japan, also could provide significant benefits. It did not take a rocket scientist to realize that combining these agents might provide a more effective treatment package than using any one of them alone. I wondered why some enterprising neuro-oncologist had not seen the potential value of the cocktail treatment strategy. I am still wondering.

ENDNOTES

1. More specifically, tamoxifen is a calmodulin antagonist. See Rowlands, M. G., et al. Comparison between inhibition of protein kinase C and antagonism of calmodulin by tamoxifen analogues. *Biochemical Pharmacology.* 1995;50(5):723-726.

2. Normal cells are inactive except when circumstances (such as injury) require them to divide for tissue growth or repair. The growth process is initiated by external biochemical signals that are incorporated into the cell nucleus via receptors on the cell membrane. In cancer cells, a proliferation of receptors leads to uncontrolled growth, sending an exaggerated signal that causes the cells to divide rapidly. The epidermal growth factor receptor is one of the most common signaling channels to be aberrant in cancer cells.

3. The prevention of angiogenesis has been widely discussed since May 1998, when the *New York Times* ran a front-page story reporting that a professor at Harvard Medical School, Dr. Judah Folkman, had developed an extraordinary new cancer treatment that completely stopped the growth of all the types of tumors on which it had been tested. The research was done entirely with mice, and cynics were quick to point out the uncertainties in translating

this research to actual clinical treatment. At the time of this writing, the jury is still out over just how effective such treatments will be; however, at least twenty drug companies are in the process of developing antiangiogenic agents, many of which are now in clinical trials.

4. Although Folkman had championed the idea of antiangiogenic drugs for almost twenty years, he had difficulty getting the funds he needed to pursue his research. Other researchers did not take the idea seriously, in part because of several false starts by Folkman in trying to establish the validity of the approach. EntreMed recognized the great potential in antiangiogenic drugs and was willing to undertake the risk of supporting Folkman's research. This is one of the finest examples of the benefits of free enterprise that I have seen. While development of antiangiogenic agents was still in an early stage, EntreMed sponsored the clinical trials with thalidomide as a "proof of principle." They later sold the rights to thalidomide to Celgene Corporation and focused their drug development program on two more powerful antiangiogenic agents, Endostatin and Angiostatin. Clinical trials involving these drugs are now in process.

5. Celgene Corporation press release. 1999 Nov 5.

6. Fine, H. A., et al. A phase-II trial of the antiangiogenic agent, thalidomide, in patients with recurrent high-grade gliomas. *Proceedings of the American Society of Clinical Oncology.* 1997;abstract 1372.

7. Glass, J., et al. Phase-I/II study of carboplatin and thalidomide in recurrent glioblastoma multiforme. *Proceedings of the American Society of Clinical Oncology.* 1999;abstract 551.

Shared Experiences

PHYSICIANS DIFFER IN HOW THEY GO ABOUT INFORMING A PATIENT THAT he or she has a fatal disease. When I had my MRI in the emergency room, the resident neurologist seemingly could not bring himself to tell me the bad news. Instead, he showed me the scan on the MRI monitor and allowed me to draw my own conclusions. When Diane and I met with Dr. Marshall a few days after my surgery, he did not downplay the seriousness of my situation, but he was quick to point out what could be done to help me, and he offered to put me in touch with patients who were long-term survivors. When we met with Dr. Chamberlain, he matter-of-factly gave us the statistics: the median survival time was less than a year, but because I was functioning at a high level, I had a good chance of surviving longer, perhaps eighteen months. When Diane pointedly asked him whether there were "stars" who did much better than anyone else, he sidestepped the question, leaving us with the impression that no one survived. Diane and I felt like we had been hit with a ton of bricks.

Our reactions to Dr. Marshall and Dr. Chamberlain were quite different. Both of them believed I would be dead in twelve to eighteen months, probably sooner, yet Dr. Marshall was quick to offer hope, while Dr. Chamberlain simply gave us the grim facts. One can argue which is the better approach. Patients are entitled to an honest appraisal of their situation, but a positive outlook, even if unrealistic, offers at least a period of time where the patient is not overwhelmed by the depressing reality of his or her disease. On the other hand, false hope will soon be dashed, perhaps resulting in even greater despair.

Anyone faced with a life-threatening illness will naturally seek out others who have survived the same disease. Even when the prognosis is abysmal, finding someone who has beaten the odds can offer hope that survival is a possibility. We may know that our chances are less than one in ten, or even one in fifty, but someone has to be that one person. Until shown otherwise, our defense mechanisms encourage us to believe that we are still in the running, that we may be among the fortunate few.

Finding a glimmer of hope, however fragile, is especially important for those afflicted with a brain tumor. Victims often are young and have no other medical problems; they are hit from out of the blue with the most crushing blow imaginable. Many learn of their tumors abruptly, often after a seizure. Others, like me, know that something is amiss but never suspect that anything could be so drastically wrong. I often joke about the horseshoe-sized scar from my craniotomy because the entire experience was very much like being kicked in the head.

The brain is the most important part of the body, the essential basis of a human being's existence. We all know people who have suffered brain damage. Whether due to injury or illness, the consequences are often devastating. Knowing that you personally have a growing tumor that will inflict such damage is an overwhelming experience. If you were a dog, you would tuck your tail between your legs and whimper.

The psychological impact of helplessness has been studied extensively. When an animal experiences a severe stressor, such as a near-drowning

SURVIVING "TERMINAL" CANCER

experience or an intense electrical shock, the effects are not confined to the immediate emotional impact of the stressor. Instead, a pattern of helplessness may ensue, causing the animal to become dysfunctional. It learns more slowly, becomes more subordinate to other animals, shows inappropriate emotional reactions, and generally appears depressed. It is as if the positive aspects of life have been overwhelmed by the stressful event. The result is that the animal's psyche appears fragile and in danger of shattering. Time can alleviate many of these reactions when the stressful event is an isolated occurrence, but repeated stress produces durable effects that are difficult to overcome. To counteract these effects, the animal must be repeatedly exposed to situations where it succeeds in avoiding future stress or obtaining positive rewards.

Humans are animals, and the laws of helplessness also apply to us. Being told we soon will die from cancer is a highly stressful event. Living with that expectation is even more debilitating. In addition to this stress, most brain tumor patients have incurred brain damage that undercuts our ability to function. We think more slowly and become confused more easily. Some of us suffer from aphasia and sensorimotor deficits. It is difficult not to feel helpless.

But humans have an advantage over other animals in that much of our learning comes from observing others. If other people can successfully battle a life-threatening tumor, then coping with our own disease is a real possibility. In other words, we can copy our fellow human beings and hope that we, too, will succeed in dealing with an otherwise overwhelming problem. And so we seek out other people who have our disease, searching for long-term survivors.

Seeking Out Survivors

Patients with primary brain tumors (as opposed to metastatic brain tumors) are relatively rare; the typical oncologist or neurologist encounters only a few of them in clinical practice. Until my diagnosis, I had known only one person with a brain tumor, a member of the UCSD administration who survived eighteen months. Even after I began treatment, I met few long-term survivors; UCSD was not among the major centers for brain tumor research, and glioblastoma patients who had a positive outcome were few and far between. Fortunately, I discovered the BrainTmr group on the Internet, which gave me access to the case histories of many different patients, not just those who had been treated by my own physicians. This made a huge difference in my outlook. I saw that there were, indeed, long-term survivors. For some patients, treatment was successful. I knew that my own chances of survival were slim, but, apart from the statistics, there was no basis for believing that my treatment could not be equally successful.

I began to follow the case histories reported to our BrainTmr group. It was clear that some participants were more aggressive in exploring every possible avenue that might lead to effective treatment. I was especially impressed by a half-dozen or so people, including two sets of parents fighting to help their children survive brain-stem gliomas, a podiatrist trying to save the life of his sister-in-law, and a German chemist trying to save his wife. All of them frequently contributed information about clinical trials as well as nontraditional treatments eschewed by the medical community. Much of this information led me to incorporate new agents into my own treatment regimen. But more important at the time were their examples. I did not have to wait and let fate take its course. Simply making an effort to cope with the situation, even if I were unsuccessful, was therapeutic. The more information I could marshal to aid my efforts to cope, the less overwhelmed I felt by my situation.

These four patients eventually succumbed to their disease, although the wife of the German chemist survived four to five years and the podiatrist's sister-in-law lived for almost eight years. In each case I felt deep sadness as well as gratitude—they had taught me a great deal, and I was determined to use the information they had shared to improve my own chances.

As I became more conversant with the medical literature on the treatment of gliomas, my participation in the BrainTmr group increased. I discovered several studies that no one else had heard about. The most surprising was the finding by an Italian group that melatonin substantially increased survival time. I was astonished that anything so benign could have such a big effect, but even more surprised that physicians in this country had not embraced the research results. Although the study was published in a major cancer journal, no one in the American neuro-oncology community seemed aware of its existence. I also reported a study by a research group in India, which found that gamma-linolenic acid infused directly into the tumor bed produced major destruction of the tumor without evident side effects. Physicians in England were using the drug to treat pancreatic cancer, and they believed oral ingestion of gamma-linolenic acid could be beneficial. I routinely passed on such information to the group.

Helping Others to Cope

Those who participate in the BrainTmr group are asked to list their diagnosis and the date it was made. This allows other participants to identify long-term survivors and inquire about the details of their treatment. Once I reached the two-year survival mark, I began to receive a large number of inquiries, so I kept a brief summary of my case history on file for those seeking information.

It occurred to me that other long-term survivors were probably receiving similar inquiries. I asked the owner of virtualtrials.com,[1] a Web site containing information about brain tumors and their treatments, if he would be interested in adding a section where long-term survivors could post their case histories. He was eager to do so, and he encouraged us to include contact information as well as pictures to personalize our stories. The result of this endeavor was an abrupt increase in the number of messages I received. Most offered congratulations on being a long-term survivor or thanks for providing an inspirational example, but several sought my opinion about various treatment options. Inquiries came from all over the world, including Norway, Australia, Ireland, Jordan, England, Israel, Canada, and Peru. I realized that the Internet had essentially destroyed geographic boundaries: people who never would have made contact in the past can now do so in a matter of seconds.

In response to these inquiries, I sent a twenty-page summary of treatment options along with a promise to try and answer any questions the patient might have. Often this led to follow-up phone conversations. I felt uneasy about playing the role of medical advisor, but as time went on and I saw more and more of the treatments prescribed by physicians, I became increasingly convinced that my advice was, in fact, valuable. At the very least, it served to counteract the uncritical acceptance of a great deal of medical advice that I considered misguided.

I received inquiries from patients outside the BrainTmr group as well, mainly friends of friends. It is supposedly a statistical fact that any two people are connected by no more than two to three common acquaintances. Each person knows hundreds of people, each of whom knows hundreds of others. This geometrical progression soon grows to include any individual you might name. Thus, a given brain tumor patient has a friend concerned for his or her welfare, and that friend may be your friend as well.

In May 1996, I ran into a friend from Drake University at a meeting of the Association for Behavior Analysis. He had survived a heart-lung transplant a couple years earlier, and we commiserated about our near-death experiences. A few weeks later, he called to ask if I would be willing to talk to a friend of his whose son had just been diagnosed with a brain tumor. The son had a low-grade oligodendroglioma, about which I knew relatively little. But I knew enough to advise him about which physicians to see, and I hoped that the advice proved useful.

A few months later I attended a meeting of the Psychonomic Society, an organization of experimental psychologists, in St. Louis.

I had several friends living there, all associated with Washington University. I learned that one of their friends, a rheumatologist, had just been diagnosed with a glioblastoma, and I agreed to contact his wife with any help I could provide. Over the next few months, she and I had numerous conversations about treatments he would not likely receive from his oncologist, including tamoxifen, Accutane, melatonin, and gamma-linolenic acid. Her husband had been hospitalized for an infection acquired at the time of his surgery, and he was unable to receive chemotherapy. His wife appreciated my advice, but his physicians were unwilling to implement the treatments I suggested. We gradually lost contact, and I learned from my friends that her husband had died soon after.

In addition to the brain tumor patients referred to me by friends, I was surprised to receive referrals from my physicians. My radiation oncologist, Dr. Hodgens, put me in touch with a San Diego man who was bedridden due to the effects of his surgery. He was an engineer by training, several years younger than I, and severely depressed. I did my best to cheer him up by explaining the many different treatment options available and providing a written description and evaluation of these treatments. I succeeded in raising his spirits, but I knew his situation was far worse than mine had ever been and did not envy the difficulties that lay ahead for him.

My most surprising referral came from my neurosurgeon, Dr. Larry Marshall. His cousin Chris lived in Alaska and had just been diagnosed with a glioblastoma. Dr. Marshall asked me to provide any information I could about nontraditional treatments. When I contacted Chris, I found that he suffered from aphasia due to his surgery, and he was terribly depressed. He preferred to have his wife, Barbara, handle most of the communication. First I suggested they go outside of Alaska to obtain better medical advice, as their physician had recommended whole-head radiation, a procedure that was rejected as standard treatment many years ago. I encouraged Barbara to contact Dr. Jay Loeffler at Harvard, one of the leading radiation oncologists in the country. Dr. Loeffler agreed with my assessment, commenting, "They don't do that anymore even in third-world countries."

I also encouraged them to adopt the "cocktail" approach to treatment, including not only tamoxifen, Accutane, and melatonin, but also thalidomide, which had recently become available. Shortly after this conversation they traveled to UCSF to get further recommendations for treatment. The physician advised Chris to receive a second operation, which had the unfortunate consequence of making him yet more aphasic. It also resulted in a case of meningitis, which delayed his treatment. Later, when Chris had recovered, UCSF adamantly refused to cooperate with the cocktail approach. Instead, the physicians convinced them to participate in a clinical trial using a new chemotherapy drug, temozolomide (Temodar), which had shown promise of being an improvement over other forms of chemotherapy.

I had been closely following the development of this drug. Experiments done with rats had indicated that temozolomide combined with BCNU produced a synergistic effect,[3] but clinical studies using temozolomide alone were somewhat disappointing. The drug produced a high initial response relative to other chemotherapy agents, but these tended to be short-lived and had little effect on overall survival time.[4] On the other hand, several members of the BrainTmr group had used the drug with some success, so I was ambivalent.

Chris and Barbara were persuaded to participate in the trial, which used temozolomide as a single agent, and they abandoned the cocktail approach. A few months later, Barbara called to say that the treatment had failed and UCSF recommended no further treatment. They had advised her to make arrangements for hospice care. Chris died shortly thereafter.

These cases were but a few of the inquiries I received. Almost all the people I advised were initially receptive to my ideas about how the disease should be addressed, yet most eventually acquiesced to the

SURVIVING "TERMINAL" CANCER

advice of their physicians, who advocated either the standard treatment or a new chemotherapy trial. But there were exceptions. One was the wife of a fellow professor at UCSD. Immediately after she was diagnosed, I received inquiries from a half-dozen people affiliated with the university about whether I could provide any help. I quickly established a relationship with the couple, describing to them my own treatment and its underlying philosophy. I found them very receptive, in part because their son became involved in our interactions. An undergraduate at Harvard, Alex seemed to have more common sense at age nineteen than most of the physicians with whom I had interacted. He immediately grasped the significance of the cocktail approach to treatment, and he proceeded to do his own research of the medical literature, with a small amount of guidance from me. This became important when the family began making the rounds of the brain tumor centers. Alex gave the physicians the third degree about their proposed treatment regimens, leaving his father to smooth the ruffled feathers. Perhaps as a result of this bad cop–good cop routine, the physicians became more receptive to the cocktail approach, although none actually agreed to use it. Ultimately, the family decided to pursue this approach on their own, using a local oncologist who was amenable to trying nonstandard treatments.

From their experience, I learned that patients who are intelligent and well-informed can shape their own treatment, but only with difficulty. Physicians respect knowledgeable people who will challenge their preconceptions, but they are nevertheless reluctant to go beyond the standard treatments. Even when a patient presents a good case for pursuing something novel and promising, it takes a great deal of perseverance and fortitude to obtain the necessary cooperation. And even the most ardent efforts do not necessarily end in success. In the case of the professor's wife, numerous complications arose that prevented the complete implementation of the treatment plan, and none of the agents used provided a beneficial effect. Sadly, she lived only slightly longer than the typical one-year period. I had feared this would be the case because her tumor continued to grow throughout radiation, which is among the worst prognostic indicators. Glioblastoma tumors, like all forms of cancer, vary in their ferocity, and some are simply unresponsive to any treatment.

For most of the patients whom I advise, there is a conflict between the physician's adherence to the standard treatment and the patient's interest in receiving the best treatment based on the latest research. Only the most intelligent and aggressive patients manage to convince their physicians to try the drug cocktail approach. Ironically, the most prestigious brain tumor centers, where oncologists are presumably best informed about cutting-edge developments, are often the most resistant to nonconventional approaches. Their recommendations seem restricted to two categories: the standard first-line treatment (aptly characterized as "slash, burn, and poison"), and participation in clinical trials that they themselves are conducting (usually investigating the effects of chemotherapy drugs that have been studied with other forms of cancer). I do my best to provide the armament patients need to question, and hopefully resist, these authoritative treatment prescriptions.

At last count, I have advised over two hundred patients—or, more often, significant others working on their behalf. These included a successful attorney in Melbourne, Australia, an engineer in Minneapolis, my aunt's minister, and the wife of an attorney in Los Angeles who worked for a good friend. I have learned something from all of them, especially in terms of how intelligent people deal with a difficult situation, and how the medical community reacts to challenges to its orthodoxy. Receiving the best possible care is not a simple endeavor. Often it requires as much energy to combat the resistance of the medical establishment as it does to fight the disease itself. This is energy that a brain tumor patient cannot afford to expend needlessly. Patients are not well served by the standard treatments currently available, but to go beyond those treatments requires patients to become informed about their own medical condition and take an active role in decision making. The medical community does its best to discourage patients from assuming an active role, and only those with exceptional spunk are able to obtain the treatment they believe to be in their best interests.

ENDNOTES

1. The Web site www.virtualtrials.com includes a listing of clinical trials by geographic region, a description of new treatments, survivor stories, and more. Al Musella, the owner of the site, also oversees a database that tries to relate treatment outcome to the specific treatments that patients receive. As I will discuss in chapter 10, such record keeping is a better way to advance knowledge about brain tumors than the current clinical trial system.

2. My summary of treatment options can be found at www.virtualtrials.com/williams.cfm. I update it annually.

3. Plowman, J., et al. Preclinical antitumor activity of temozolomide in mice: efficacy against human brain tumor zenographs and synergism with 1, 3-bis (2-chloroethyl)-1 nitrosourea. *Cancer Research*. 1994;54(14):3793-3799.

4. Newlands, E. S., et al. The Charing Cross Hospital experience with temozolomide in patients with gliomas. *European Journal of Cancer*. 1996;32A(13):2236-2241.

A System in Need of Reform

SECTION TWO

THE CURRENT MEDICAL SYSTEM DOES NOT PROVIDE THE BEST POSSIBLE treatment for cancer patients, and especially not for those with brain tumors. In my own case, I would likely be dead if I had followed the advice of my neuro-oncologist. My prognosis was dismal. Only a tiny fraction of glioblastoma patients are long-term survivors: estimates range from 1 or 2 percent (based on government statistics) to 3 to 5 percent (for those participating in clinical trials at major brain tumor centers). Of these, the great majority are much younger than I was at the time of my diagnosis. Moreover, my tumor was extremely large, there was a substantial amount of residual tumor after surgery, and radiation left my tumor unchanged in size. Each of these facts reduced the likelihood that I would be a survivor. I am convinced I would not have survived had I not pursued "unproven" treatments in addition to the standard treatments I received. Neuro-oncologists routinely oppose the use of "unproven" treatments, an attitude that seriously diminishes their patients' chances of survival.

Of course, the few successful glioblastoma outcomes, including my own, could be due to any number of factors. Tumors are idiosyncratic; some may respond to any treatment, while others may grow rapidly regardless of treatment. The outcome of any treatment regimen is probabilistic—there is no guarantee that it will work for a particular patient. Indeed, the standard treatments typically recommended by neuro-oncologists—radiation and chemotherapy—have a very low success rate.

Rather than simply accept this small chance of success, a patient is better advised to look beyond the standard protocol for additional treatments. Different treatments have different mechanisms of action, and the laws of probability imply that the more treatments a patient uses, the greater the chances that at least one of them will succeed. Moreover, even small effects from individual treatments may have a cumulative benefit. Therefore, by combining as many different treatments as possible without creating life-threatening toxicities, patients may improve their chances of survival.

In the following pages, I do not wish to demean the competence of physicians, especially neuro-oncologists and neurosurgeons. These specialists are highly intelligent and highly trained. Neurosurgery is generally regarded as the most prestigious branch of surgery, and only the most talented medical students complete the rigorous training involved. Neuro-oncology demands more training than virtually any other non-surgical specialty, as it requires separate residencies in both oncology and neurology in addition to special training in neuro-oncology itself. Furthermore, neuro-oncologists work with patients who have very poor prospects, and the grim outcomes must be depressing to observe. Given the training, expertise, and long hours required, physicians are underpaid. This is especially true for physicians who have spent an additional three to five years of residency to become experts in their specialties, which means they are often in their mid-thirties and deep in debt before they can begin their medical practice.

Despite the high regard I have for physicians who treat cancer patients, the following chapters will be highly critical of the way neuro-oncologists function. I do not question any physician's personality or competence; instead, I argue that physician training and the way cancer treatment is institutionalized often are not in the patient's best interest. I also argue that governmental policies reinforce and perpetuate a flawed medical system.

Conventions of the Medical System
and Their Ramifications

CHAPTER SEVEN

FOR EVERY DISEASE THERE IS A GOLD STANDARD OF TREATMENT THAT clinical trials have shown to be more effective than other treatments. Physicians who ignore the evidence produced by these trials and instead use only their clinical experience are deemed unscientific, if not incompetent. They may also be accused of opportunism, because the "unproven treatments" they recommend are often accompanied by mail solicitations and other marketing efforts that appear economically motivated.

No one can argue against using the scientific method to establish rigorous medical standards. Judgments based on clinical observation alone can be deceptive due to the placebo effect, imprecise or subjective measurements, selective attention to cases that confirm one's expectations, and other factors. Some clinical misjudgments can be astounding. My favorite example is that of Dr. Antonio Moniz, who was awarded the Nobel Prize for Medicine in 1949 for his development of the frontal lobotomy as a treatment for schizophrenia. Despite the devastating deficits produced by the frontal lobotomy, physicians persisted in using this barbaric procedure for two decades, citing their subjective observation that it improved patient behavior.

While clinical trials are sometimes necessary to eliminate mistakes in medical practice, using them as the sole criterion for determining which treatments are available can reduce a patient's chance of survival. This is especially true when the gold standard of treatment is only minimally successful. For most cancer treatments, "minimal success" is an apt description,[1] but even minimal success cannot be claimed for glioblastoma treatments. It is imperative to explore new alternatives, yet patients are discouraged from doing so. To understand why, it is necessary to examine the approval process that governs the availability of treatment.

The Clinical Trial Process

For a new treatment to be marketed, it must be approved by the FDA. The approval process involves a set of clinical trials, usually consisting of three phases. Phase-I trials are intended to establish the safety profile of the drug and the dosages that optimize the cost-benefit ratio. Typically, phase-I trials involve only a few patients, and trial outcomes are not published. Phase-II trials involve more patients, usually thirty to one hundred, and are intended to demonstrate treatment efficacy. Often the trials are restricted to individual treatment centers and are unavailable elsewhere. For this reason, participants may not represent random samples of the patient population. Phase-II clinical trials must provide evidence that treatments have some efficacy in order to justify further investigation in phase-III clinical trials.

Phase-III trials are much larger in scope and usually involve several different research centers.[2] Patients are randomly assigned to a treatment group or a control group, with each group having an equivalent set of subjects. Patients in the control group may be given no treatment, a placebo, or an established treatment that may provide at

SURVIVING "TERMINAL" CANCER

least some benefit. The mean or median outcome for patients in the treatment group is compared to the outcome for patients in the control group (who are not receiving the experimental treatment). If a treatment demonstrates a statistically significant improvement, it is certified by the FDA. Physicians typically will not prescribe a treatment unless it is FDA approved.

The Economics of Drug Research

Because the effect of a treatment is highly variable among trial participants, a phase-III trial typically requires a large number of patients.[3] For this reason, phase-III trials are expensive. The National Cancer Institute sponsors some of these trials, but increasingly the costs are assumed by drug companies hoping to receive FDA approval for their products. As a result, drugs that are potentially profitable are far more likely to be studied in clinical trials. An agent that is not patentable or that is already available for purposes other than cancer treatment will almost never become the subject of a phase-III clinical trial, unless the National Cancer Institute sponsors it.

Many promising agents have not been certified by the clinical trial process and consequently have been ignored as treatment options. In an earlier chapter I described my attempts to interest my own physicians, the American Brain Tumor Association, and others in the substantial data supporting the efficacy of both melatonin (studied in Italy) and gamma-linolenic acid (tested in India), but ultimately my efforts were fruitless. I have yet to see a single American oncologist incorporate either of these agents into his or her treatment protocol, despite the fact that neither has any identifiable toxicity to normal cells.

American oncologists have little interest in treatments developed outside the United States, yet they eagerly develop new clinical trials for American chemotherapy agents, the great majority of which have been established for other forms of cancer.[4] (The platinum drugs, for example, were first used for testicular cancer but later adapted to many other cancers as well.) Clinical trials for established chemotherapy agents require far less bureaucratic oversight than those involving completely new treatments, because the drugs being studied have already received FDA approval for cancer.

The fact that an agent has never been tested in a phase-III trial does not mean it is ineffective. The economics of drug development are a more powerful determinant of what gets studied than whether there are plausible grounds for believing a given agent might be efficacious. Nevertheless, treatments that have not reached phase-III clinical trials are typically considered "unproven." Such treatments are viewed with suspicion and are rarely used, even if there is reason to believe they will improve a patient's outcome.

Proven vs. Unproven Treatments

The rigid distinction between proven and unproven treatments is a fundamental problem in cancer treatment today. Lumped together in the "unproven" category are treatments from alternative medicine, treatments developed in other countries, and agents that have been subjected to phase-II clinical trials but have not advanced to phase III. All of these have the same status as far as conventional medicine is concerned. Even when a phase-II trial suggests that a treatment may be effective, it often is largely ignored.

For glioblastoma and other fatal diseases, none of the "proven" treatments offers a significant hope for survival. Moreover, there is reason to believe that a number of unproven treatments are at least as effective and substantially less toxic than the proven treatments, yet these are withheld from patients simply because they are not FDA certified. Oncologists typically will not prescribe unproven treatments outside of clinical trials, and very few will inform their patients about promising results generated in phase-II trials. First, an oncologist is unlikely to advise a patient that another oncologist has a better treatment for his or her cancer. Second, oncologists conducting their own clinical trials must compete with physicians at other institutions for suitable trial subjects. Finally, because of contractual obligations to drug companies that fund these trials, once a trial has been initiated, it often must be completed regardless of how well it is going. Physicians may be aware of extremely promising trials being conducted at other institutions, but they will not volunteer this information because they need patients for their own research. This failure to inform patients may occur even when another physician's trial has been completed and considerable information exists about the potential benefits of the experimental treatment.

An example from my own experience concerns Accutane, a drug that is FDA-approved for the treatment of acne. Its chemical name is isotretinoin, also known as 13-*cis*-retinoic acid; it is a first cousin of trans-retinoic acid, which is used in the treatment of cancer, especially in children. (It is also the active ingredient in the skin medication Retin-A.) Isotretinoin is an acid form of vitamin A. Unlike regular vitamin A, vitamin A acid is not stored in the liver. This greatly reduces the chance of liver toxicity caused by high dosages of vitamin A, which can be fatal. Although I had known about clinical trials testing whether vitamin A could prevent cancer (ironically, beta-carotene, the precursor to vitamin A, turned out to actually increase the risk of cancer), I had no inkling that it was actively being investigated for brain cancer and was producing positive results. Only by chance did I see a passing comment made by Dr. Victor Levin, perhaps the leading neuro-oncologist in the country, of the M.D. Anderson Cancer Center at the University of Texas. When Dr. Levin was asked by a member of our BrainTmr group for his opinion about tamoxifen and other new treatments that seemed considerably less toxic than standard chemotherapy, he mentioned that Accutane was similarly nontoxic and that they had just finished a successful phase-II clinical trial using it to treat glioblastoma. I found an abstract of the study in *Proceedings of the American Society of Clinical Oncology,* which showed that the drug produced tumor regression or stabilization in 45 percent of the trial patients.[5] I then contacted Dr. William Yung, Levin's colleague at M.D. Anderson, for additional information. Combining the two resources, I was able to determine the dosages and administration schedule used in the study. On the basis of this meager information, I decided to add the drug to my own treatment regimen. Desperate to increase my chances of survival, I traveled to Tijuana to obtain it on my own. But because I had already created friction with Dr. Chamberlain over my use of tamoxifen and my possible participation in Dr. Friedman's monoclonal antibody trial, I decided not to tell him about the Accutane until much later.[6]

Dr. Chamberlain had, in fact, known about the Accutane trial from its inception. He had done his training in neuro-oncology under Dr. Levin, and the two men were still in contact. Shortly after my first clean MRI, I told Dr. Chamberlain that I had been taking Accutane. He seemed pleased, commenting about what a nice study Drs. Levin and Yung had conducted. I found it remarkable that I would not have learned about the drug if I had not been lucky enough to see Dr. Levin's comment to the BrainTmr Internet group. Here was a low-toxicity treatment that was shown to have a significant beneficial effect—one that apparently could be combined with other treatments—yet the only patients who had access to it were those at M.D. Anderson. The only reason I was able to obtain it on my own was because I could purchase it in Mexico without a prescription.

Both Accutane and tamoxifen are now prescribed by a small minority of neuro-oncologists throughout the country, and thalidomide is also beginning to be used with some frequency. This is due, in part, to patients finding information on their own, often from Internet resources such as our BrainTmr group, and demanding access to these treatments. Both tamoxifen and Accutane are certified for other medical conditions, and thalidomide was recently approved for the treatment of leprosy.

Legally, any of these drugs can be prescribed for any purpose at a physician's discretion. This is known as "off-label use."

As possible brain tumor treatments, thalidomide, tamoxifen, and Accutane have been subjected only to phase-II clinical trials. It is unlikely that they will ever be studied in phase-III cancer trials because they are already FDA-approved for other indications. For a drug company to invest the considerable money required for additional phase-III trials, it must believe that the market for a new indication is substantial. Glioblastomas are relatively rare, and the market incentive is too weak to justify the expense. Because these drugs are not specifically approved for brain tumors, few neuro-oncologists are willing to use them despite evidence of efficacy in phase-II trials. As a result, most patients never learn about these treatments.

Restricted Access

Restricting the availability of new drugs is especially troublesome when they are known to have minimal toxicity. As argued in chapter 5, tamoxifen, Accutane, thalidomide, gamma-linolenic acid, and other agents are prime candidates for drug cocktails analogous to those that have revolutionized the treatment of AIDS. By not acknowledging the potential clinical value of these agents, the issue of a cocktail approach to brain tumor treatment is not even broached. Even when patients express a strong desire to try drug combinations, they are almost always opposed by their oncologists. Only the most persevering patient is likely to find a physician who is willing to prescribe experimental drug combinations. After the standard treatments fail, which they typically do, clinical trials may be an option, but even these do not offer drug cocktails. In recent trials, a new chemotherapy agent called Temodar was combined with other treatments. This was an improvement over the one-drug-at-a-time approach, but it was still far from the cocktail philosophy.

Oncologists rarely deviate from conventional treatments, even upon a patient's request. There is no valid scientific basis for this refusal. The fact is, standard treatments for brain tumor patients are little more than a death sentence. To refuse access to promising alternatives simply because they are unproven, even when such alternatives are legal according to FDA rules, may be in accord with accepted medical practice, but it is a gross violation of any acceptable ethical principle. It is the patient's life that is in dire jeopardy. If the physician can offer no more than a few more months' survival time, it should be the patient's prerogative to choose experimental treatments that seem more promising. Opposing that choice because the unproven treatments might be harmful to the patient is incredibly presumptuous on the part of the physician, especially when the unproven treatments are shown to be far less toxic than the standard treatments.

If an oncologist were in the same position as the patient, what treatment would he or she choose? I believe that most physicians would consider every feasible option, either alone or in combination with other agents, and anything else that might increase the odds of survival. Whether drugs were FDA-approved for brain tumors would not be a consideration. More critical would be the odds of treatment success given the current state of knowledge, and the trade-off between those odds and the risks of undergoing the treatment.

But the typical patient is offered only a Hobson's choice. On the one hand are the standard treatments that offer little hope of significantly extending survival time. On the other are clinical trials that are often motivated by considerations other than the greatest likelihood of treatment efficacy. But now, in the age of the Internet, communication among patients allows access to information about existing clinical trials as well as any preliminary results. Many physicians are not pleased with this development, because it means the authority of their treatment recommendations will be challenged. This is as it should be, given the lack of success for the great majority of cancer patients who have followed those recommendations.

ENDNOTES

1. Although the overall success rate of cancer treatment, especially with respect to metastatic cancer, has improved only minimally over the past three decades, there have been notable successes, including the multiple drug approach to childhood leukemia, radiation and chemotherapy for Hodgkin's disease, and the use of platinum compounds in the treatment of testicular cancer.

2. The most elaborate phase-III clinical trials involve double-blind studies, where neither the patient nor the physician knows if the patient is assigned to the treatment or control group. This practice is intended to eliminate bias due to expectations of the patient or physician. For many medical problems, such as depression, double-blind studies are essential because the measures of treatment efficacy are somewhat subjective, and because patients may improve simply because of positive expectations. Cancer, however, is unlikely to be susceptible to the placebo effect. And, given the high incidence of side effects for cancer treatments, few clinicians will fail to recognize which patients are in the treatment group and which are in the control. If a patient is vomiting all over the clinic, he or she is likely in the treatment group.

The procedures used in double-blind studies hinder clinicians from monitoring a treatment's progress. Results are analyzed only at periodic intervals, so patients in the control group cannot receive the treatment until very late in the game, even if the treatment is highly effective. Accordingly, some people consider double-blind trials unethical for diseases that are unlikely to be influenced by the placebo effect. The essential feature of a phase-III trial is that subjects are randomly assigned to different treatment groups, not that clinicians know to which group a patient is assigned.

3. Patient outcome varies widely, and it is impossible to know whether individual results are due to the treatment or to other factors (such as age or level of functioning prior to treatment). Because a trial's outcome will include variability due to any number of factors, statistical analysis is required to separate the true effect of the treatment from the effects of other variables. Many clinical trials will use large numbers of subjects in an attempt to cancel out the unwanted variation and isolate the effect of the treatment.

4. For glioblastoma treatments, the great majority of clinical trials follow a well-trodden path, testing chemotherapy agents that are effective in treating other forms of cancer. Such trials have repeatedly shown minimal beneficial effects, in terms of both the percentage of patients who show tumor reduction

and the duration of any positive responses that occur. While there may be occasional exceptions, this approach to clinical trial research—trying yet more variations of chemotherapy—has been an unquestionable failure. The only reason it persists is because the clinical trial system is economically driven.

5. Yung, W. K., et al. Treatment of recurrent malignant gliomas with high-dose 13-*cis*-retinoic acid. *Clinical Cancer Research.* 1996;2(12):1931-1935.

6. Self-prescription can be risky in terms of potential side effects and drug interactions. But because Accutane was already used for other purposes, I found a great deal of information about its potential toxicities and contraindications in the *Physicians Desk Reference (PDR),* the well-known pharmaceutical reference used by physicians. I determined that the threat posed by my glioblastoma loomed larger than the risks from the drug itself.

Cancer patients are well advised to tell their oncologists about all the medications they are taking. Adverse drug interactions frequently occur with prescription drugs and various supplements. Moreover, drugs often have potential side effects that need monitoring. For example, Accutane does have occasional liver toxicity, so liver enzyme tests are needed to ensure that such toxicity is minimized. Unfortunately, cancer patients are often afraid to provide complete information to their oncologists because of the opposition they typically encounter.

Arbitrary Policies Exclude
Promising Treatments

CHAPTER EIGHT

UNLESS A DRUG RECEIVES FDA APPROVAL, ONCOLOGISTS TYPICALLY will not prescribe it outside of clinical trials. Few patients will learn about the drug, and even fewer will be able to obtain it. This is especially unfortunate when a drug has shown potent beneficial effects. Because of the overwhelming importance of FDA certification, it is essential to look closely at the FDA's criteria for approval.

Arbitrary Statistical Requirements

The goal of a phase-III trial is to show that a treatment produces a statistically significant difference between the treatment and control group. A "statistically significant difference" means that the result was so unlikely to have occurred by chance that we would expect it to occur again if we repeated the experiment.

All scientific measurement involves some degree of chance, or experimental error, which is to say that results will vary when an experiment is replicated. Such variability arises from numerous sources, but, in general, the greater the number of variables that are not explicitly controlled, the greater the amount of error. In clinical trials, the more that patients vary in their individual characteristics (such as age or Karnofsky score), the greater the variability in outcome for reasons other than the treatment. If patients are similar in almost every respect, there will likely be a small degree of error.

Consider a hypothetical clinical trial involving one hundred brain tumor patients, ages twenty to eighty. Researchers want to know if an experimental treatment increases average survival time. Because age affects survival time, the trial results show a great deal of variation— some patients live for weeks, others live for years. It is difficult to know if the average survival time was due to the treatment, the variability in patient age, or a combination. If a second clinical trial were conducted involving patients with a different distribution of ages, the results from the first trial might or might not be replicated.

Participants in a clinical trial differ along many dimensions other than age, including tumor type, response to radiation, and Karnofsky score (a number ranging from 10 to 100 that indicates the degree of functional deficits; 100 equals no deficits). Some of these differences are not well understood. For example, people with different genetic profiles have different susceptibilities to cancer and different sensitivities to treatment agents. Given the enormous variability among clinical trial participants, trial results that are better than the norm might be due to this patient variability rather than the effect of the treatment.

In an effort to see the true results of the treatment under study, clinicians take steps to reduce the ambiguity of interpretation caused by this variability. For example, they use a large number of trial participants, and they randomly assign patients to either a treatment or control group. The larger the number of patients, the more likely it is that age, genetics, and other "confounding variables" will be similarly distributed across the two groups. The idea is to make the two groups as similar as possible with respect to all variables except the treatment itself. Thus, if the groups show a difference in average survival time (or other measures of patient outcome), the effect can be ascribed to the experimental treatment.

Of course, variability may still occur within a treatment or control group, so it is still possible that a trial's results are due to chance. To assert that results actually reflect the effects of the experimental treatment, researchers must demonstrate that the difference in outcome between the treatment and control groups is statistically significant—that there is a low probability the effect is due to random error. What is a low probability? The conventional level, which is used by the FDA, is less than .05 (5 percent, or a one in twenty chance that the result is due to random error). Therefore, to receive FDA approval, a treatment must have a .05 level of statistical significance.

This .05 level is arbitrary. At one time in my own field of experimental psychology, the professional journals adopted a much more stringent criterion of .01. As a result, many experiments that would have produced a statistically significant effect using the .05 criterion failed to do so at .01, even though differences in outcome between experimental and control groups remained unchanged. These experiments were never published, although their findings were almost certainly true and replicable.

The .05 level of statistical significance, which is required for FDA approval, is entirely a matter of convention. Nevertheless, it is a barrier that must be overcome before new treatments are made available to patients. No matter how promising a treatment may be, the FDA will not approve it unless it meets this statistical criterion. This has important implications for clinical practice. For example, a recent phase-III clinical trial conducted in Canada involved brachytherapy, the procedure in which radioactive iodine seeds are temporarily implanted in the tumor area.[1] A published abstract stated that there was no reliable increase in survival time as a result of the procedure. A patient reading only this conclusion would likely avoid the procedure, especially given its significant side effects. But a closer reading revealed that brachytherapy resulted in a longer median survival time relative to the control group, though the difference only attained the .07 level of statistical significance. In other words, because there was a 7 percent chance that the trial results were due to random error, the researchers reported no therapeutic effect.

For brain cancer and other diseases that currently have no effective treatment, it would make sense to lower this barrier of statistical significance, allowing more treatments to become available. For example, if conventional medicine adopted the .20 level of probability, many more treatments would be eligible for FDA certification. True, there would be a 20 percent chance that trial results were due to random variability, but for brain tumors and other fatal diseases, this seems an acceptable risk in order to gain access to promising new treatments.

One of the first lessons that students learn in any statistics class is the danger of accepting the "null hypothesis." When an experiment fails to meet a criterion of statistical significance, such as the .05 level, this does not prove that no effect exists. It shows only that a reliable difference has not been demonstrated in terms of the statistical barrier agreed upon before undertaking the experiment. Had a less rigorous statistical criterion been used, a very different conclusion might have been reached.

The medical community, in league with the FDA, has virtually fallen in love with the null hypothesis. As a result, many potential treatments have been taken off the table even though they are likely to be effective—perhaps more effective than currently available treatments.

Arbitrary Control Conditions

The statistical criterion for FDA approval is not the only arbitrary practice in the certification process. Control conditions, which are negotiated by the FDA and clinical trial investigators, vary widely from trial to trial. Because phase-III clinical trials assign subjects to experimental and control groups, it is critical that the control condition be selected judiciously. A new treatment may appear effective when compared to a placebo, but ineffective when compared to an already existing treatment.

In 1996, for example, the FDA approved the first new brain tumor treatment in over twenty years, Gliadel. Gliadel consists of polymer wafers, containing BCNU, which are placed inside the tumor cavity at the time of surgery. FDA approval was based on a clinical trial in which patients with recurrent high-grade tumors were randomly assigned to receive either Gliadel wafers or placebo wafers.[2] The median survival time after treatment was thirty-one weeks for the Gliadel group, and twenty-three weeks for the placebo group. Survival rates six months after the treatment were 56 percent for the Gliadel group and 36 percent for the placebo group. Both of these effects were statistically significant; however, had Gliadel been compared with an existing treatment rather than a placebo, a statistically significant difference may not have occurred, and the drug may not have received FDA approval.[3]

Consider the history of temozolomide (Temodar), a new chemotherapy agent developed in England to treat grade-III and -IV gliomas. At the time of this writing, temozolomide has received FDA approval for the treatment of grade-III gliomas, but not for glioblastomas. The basis for the latter decision was a phase-III clinical trial in which temozolomide was compared with procarbazine, a chemotherapy agent commonly used as a second-line treatment when the initial treatment (nitrosoureas such as BCNU) has failed.[4] Trial participants—glioblastoma patients whose tumors had recurred—found temozolomide easier to tolerate because it was less toxic. Three additional measures were assessed: the percentage of patients who had no tumor progression for at least six months after initiation of treatment (21 percent for temozolomide vs. 9 percent for procarbazine); the median time between the start of treatment and tumor progression (2.9 months vs.

1.9 months); and the median survival time after treatment initiation (7.3 months vs. 5.8 months). The first two differences were statistically significant using the .05 criterion. The third comparison produced a statistical outcome with a probability level above .05. Despite the positive findings, the FDA determined that temozolomide did not meet its criteria for approval because the difference in survival time failed to reach the .05 statistical criterion. Had temozolomide been compared to a placebo, as Gliadel was, it most likely would have been approved for glioblastoma treatment.

Procarbazine, which was grandfathered without clinical trial certification, is still widely used without FDA interference. Given that temozolomide is clearly better in several respects, it is hard to understand why the FDA would fail to sanction temozolomide as an alternative treatment. In actual fact, the FDA's refusal to approve temozolomide for glioblastoma treatment has had minimal impact. Because the drug has been approved for grade-III gliomas,[5] it can be prescribed for other purposes as well. Oncologists now prescribe temozolomide for all types of gliomas, ignoring the distinction made by the FDA.

An Irrational System

For most cancer patients, the statistical reliability of a clinical trial is far less relevant than the measurable effects of the treatment—what percentage of patients were helped by the treatment, how long they survived, and so forth. Consider a hypothetical choice a glioblastoma patient might confront: On the one hand is a treatment thoroughly tested in a large, phase-III clinical trial. The treatment received FDA approval after it was shown to increase average survival time by one to five months when compared to a placebo. On the other hand is a new treatment, tested in a phase-II trial with fifty patients, that was shown to produce a three-year survival rate of 50 percent. (Typically, the three-year survival rate for glioblastoma patients is 10 percent.) Which treatment should the patient choose?

Neuro-oncologists playing by the rules of accepted clinical practice would prescribe the former treatment because it has received FDA approval and is believed to produce a reliable effect. The patient, however, would likely choose the experimental treatment. Though the first option is statistically reliable, a three-month increase in average survival time doesn't offer much hope for surviving the disease. The magnitude of the effects reported in the phase-II trial seems more promising, though of course there is uncertainty in choosing the unproven treatment. True, the outcome of the phase-II trial was based on a small number of patients and was not compared to a control group; however, given the dramatic improvement in average survival time, it is likely that the experimental treatment has at least some beneficial effects. Sound judgment can occur without the help of statistical analysis.

Because the FDA's statistical criteria often do not correspond to meaningful improvements in patient outcome, and because control conditions used in clinical trials are arbitrary (why was a placebo control adequate for Gliadel but not for temozolomide?), the dichotomy between approved and unapproved treatments must be considered arbitrary as well. At the very least, it should not discourage oncologists from considering agents that are supported only by phase-II data. Yet it does, and this limits the treatments available to patients who already have very few options.

Consider, too, that standard glioblastoma treatments (chemotherapy, brachytherapy, and radiosurgery) have been used since the 1970s, predating current requirements for FDA approval. According to criteria that the FDA applies to new treatment agents, none of these "standard" agents have been shown convincingly to be more effective than radiation alone.[6] If they were introduced as new glioblastoma treatments today, they would likely not receive FDA certification. Yet, they are routinely recommended despite their significant toxic effects, especially in the case of brachytherapy. Their acceptance as standard treatments is due not to supposedly rigorous FDA procedures, but to the grandfathering of existing treatments at the time that FDA requirements became more stringent, and to a nebulous consensus among neuro-oncologists based on a combination of clinical observation and phase-II clinical trials.

To patients with high-grade gliomas, the current system of medical care is irrational. First, promising new treatments are often rejected because of statistical data related to a trial's replicability—not the magnitude of a treatment's effects. Second, the standard treatments typically prescribed are highly toxic, and their efficacy is not supported by the level of evidence required for new treatments. Many agents studied in phase-II trials seem to offer at least the same benefits as traditional agents, but without the high toxicity. From a patient's perspective, it is foolish to choose standard treatments that have little evidence of success when experimental treatments show more promise. If given the choice, most patients would opt for a treatment that has not yet been shown a failure.

Making an Informed Decision

Of course, some patients do receive significant benefits from traditional treatments. A small minority of glioblastoma patients (in the range of 1 to 5 percent) will be "cured," meaning they will survive longer than five years. A much larger percentage (15 to 25 percent) will increase their survival time. Typically, these patients respond to a few rounds of chemotherapy, but their tumors begin to grow again after developing resistance to the treatment. Nevertheless, survival time may increase from fifteen to twenty-four months, whereas patients who do not respond to chemotherapy generally live four to twelve months.

Most experimental treatments follow a similar pattern. Some patients respond favorably at first, but the great majority relapse after developing a resistance to the treatment. It is difficult to know exactly what percentage of glioblastoma patients would respond to a particular experimental treatment, given that phase-II clinical trials usually do not continue long enough to assess overall survival times. Nevertheless, some pertinent data are available:

- Tamoxifen used for recurrent, high-grade gliomas was shown to cause tumor regression or stabilization in 25 to 45 percent of patients participating in a trial.[7] At least some of these patients have survived from two to eight years.
- When tamoxifen was combined with radiation and BCNU, the median survival time was sixty-nine weeks. More impressively, the two-year survival rate was 45 percent and the three-year survival rate was 24 percent.[8]
- For Accutane, the median survival time exceeded one year among patients with recurrent tumors, whereas the typical outcome with chemotherapy is three to five months.[9]
- For thalidomide, 50 percent of patients with recurrent tumors showed regression or stabilization upon initial exposure to the treatment.[10]
- A subsequent study that combined thalidomide with carboplatin increased the initial response rate to 67 percent.[11]

Regardless of the statistical reliability of these numbers, a pattern emerges. The experimental treatments appear no less effective than FDA-approved treatments, although such comparisons are suspect because of variability in subject populations.

Neuro-oncologists are acutely aware of the limitations of the standard treatment options. That is why they encourage patients to serve as guinea pigs in new clinical trials. Given the bleak prospect of success using the standard treatment options, trials are an appealing alternative. They at least offer hope that the research will lead to more effective treatments in the future, and that something positive might come out of a patient's tragedy.

But there is a third alternative for brain tumor patients: use the evidence from phase-II clinical trials to make a best-bet gamble about which combination of agents will provide the best chance for survival.

In other words, put all the treatment possibilities from phase-II trials on the table. By comparing measures of clinical efficacy—the percentage of patients whose tumors regress; the time before regrowth; the percentage of patients alive at six, twelve, eighteen, and twenty-four months—patients can make informed decisions (with the understanding that much of the evidence may be confounded by variables such as unrepresentative patient populations or bias due to subject self-selection). Why are patients not given this opportunity?

"Do No Harm"

The answer to this question ultimately harks back to the Hippocratic oath, which is believed to provide the first principle of medical practice: "do no harm."[12] In essence, it is an allegiance to this principle that discourages physicians from prescribing a treatment unless there is a professional consensus that the treatment will be effective. The assumption is that medicine is a collective enterprise that establishes approved standards of care. Physicians may not rely on their own unscientific biases as the basis for medical treatment.

As a first principle of medicine, "do no harm" has justification, but it is fundamentally inadequate when dealing with patients who have an incurable disease. When the accepted standard of care offers little hope, it is unacceptable to restrict the availability of other medical options. The prescription of only certified treatments reflects a misguided distinction in the medical community: sins of commission vs. sins of omission. If a physician does something to a patient that causes harm, the physician is more culpable than if he or she withholds a treatment that could have helped. This is a pragmatic concern that every physician must endure. Unfortunately, the consequences of restricting the availability of promising treatments can be tragic for the patient.

A physician's refusal to offer promising new treatments simply because they have not been FDA certified cannot be justified by the "do no harm" principle of medicine. Patients are entitled to promising treatments regardless of the conventions of the FDA and the medical guild. A government policy is needed to differentiate between the treatments of curable and incurable diseases. Physicians should be free to explore promising treatments from phase-II clinical trials without threat of legal action. When a patient's situation is hopeless, both patient and physician must be allowed a no-holds-barred approach to treatment.

There are risks in choosing treatments based only on their effects in phase-II clinical trials. But such risks need to be evaluated in the context of what it means to be a terminally ill patient. Because the standard treatments will fail for all but a tiny minority, the only option is to try new treatments, even if there is a possibility that these, too, will fail. Patients need to assess the evidence reported by phase-II clinical trials— hopefully with the help of their physicians—and make their best bet for what is most promising. And physicians must not interfere with their patients' decisions.

It is the patient's life that is at stake, and so it should be the patient's prerogative to assess the merits of a treatment and the trade-offs between possible risks and benefits. There can be no justification for impeding a patient's efforts to make the best gamble possible for saving his or her life.

ENDNOTES

1. Laperriere, N. J., et al. Randomized study of brachytherapy in the initial management of patients with malignant astrocytoma. *International Journal of Radiation Oncology, Biology, Physics.* 1996;41(5):1005-1011.

2. Brem, H., et al. Placebo-controlled trial of safety and efficacy of intraoperative controlled delivery by biodegradable polymers of chemotherapy for recurrent gliomas. The Polymer-Brain Tumor Treatment Group. *Lancet.* 1995;345(8956):1008-1012.

3. It is unclear whether Gliadel treatment is superior to intravenous BCNU. Indeed, there is reason to believe that the difference, if any, is minimal. The clinical trial showed that both groups had nearly the same survival rate one year after treatment, indicating that the beneficial effects of Gliadel are relatively short-term in nature. It should also be noted that two-thirds of subjects in the Gliadel trial had been diagnosed with glioblastoma and one-third with other brain tumors, so the survival times reported were somewhat inflated for glioblastoma patients. These observations are not intended to devalue Gliadel as a treatment option. Gliadel does not create the systemic side effects typically produced by intravenous BCNU, and this is no small matter. But it would be a mistake for glioblastoma patients to believe that Gliadel is a significant improvement in brain tumor treatment that will greatly increase his or her chances of survival.

4. Yung, W. K. A., et al. Randomized trial of Temodar versus procarbazine (PCB) in glioblastoma at first release. *Proceedings of the American Society for Clinical Oncology.* 1999;abstract 532.

5. Yung, W. K., et al. Multicenter phase-II trial of temozolomide in patients with anaplastic astrocytoma or anaplastic oligoastrocytoma at first relapse. Temodar Brain Tumor Group. *Journal of Clinical Oncology.* 1999;17(9):2762-2771.

6. Recently, a large phase-III clinical trial in Great Britain reported that there was no advantage in using radiation plus PCV versus radiation alone. (Brada, M., et al. Medical research council [MRC] randomized trial of adjuvant chemotherapy in high grade glioma [HGG]. *Proceedings of the American Society for Clinical Oncology.* 1998;abstract 1543.) Other trials have shown some positive effects, although these have varied from trial to trial. A meta-analysis (a controversial statistical procedure used for aggregating different experimental studies) of the numerous clinical trials involving chemotherapy concluded that there was a one-to-three-month increase in survival time when chemotherapy was added to radiation. (Fine, H. A., et al. Meta-analysis of radiation therapy with and without adjuvant chemotherapy for malignant gliomas in adults. *Cancer.* 1993;71[8]:2585-2597.) A number of retrospective analyses have also made a case for chemotherapy. Whatever the validity of this conclusion, it is important to recognize that the method used to establish it would not provide an acceptable basis for FDA approval at the present time.

7. Couldwell, W. T., et al. Clinical and radiographic response in a minority of patients with recurrent malignant gliomas treated with high-dose tamoxifen. *Neurosurgery.* 1993;32(3):485-489.

8. Vertosick, F. T., and Selker, R. G. The treatment of newly diagnosed glioblastoma multiforme using high dose tamoxifen, radiotherapy, and conventional chemotherapy. *Proceedings of the American Association of Cancer Research.* 1997;abstract 2887.

9. Yung, W. K., et al. Treatment of recurrent malignant gliomas with high-dose 13-*cis*-retinoic acid. *Clinical Cancer Research.* 1996;2(12):1931-1935.

10. See chapter 5, note 6.

11. Glass, J., et al. Phase-I/II study of carboplatin and thalidomide in recurrent glioblastoma multiforme. *Proceedings of the American Society for Clinical Oncology.* 1999;abstract 551.

12. In fact, the Hippocratic oath does not include the phrase "do no harm." The phrase appears in other writings of Hippocrates, most notably "Of the Epidemics," but the oath itself stipulates only that the physician abstain from whatever is "deleterious and mischievous." Those taking the oath swear to impart their knowledge only to their children, to the children of their teachers, and to disciples sworn to maintain the secrets of medicine. In other words, the oath provides the basis for medicine being a guild that restricts its secrets and its power only to those who have been initiated:

"I swear by Apollo the physician, and Aesculapius, and Health, and Allheal, and all the gods and goddesses, that, according to my ability and judgment, I will keep this Oath and this stipulation—to reckon him who taught me this Art equally dear to me as my parents, to share my substance with him, and relieve his necessities if required; to look upon his offspring in the same footing as my own brothers, and to teach them this art, if they shall wish to learn it, without fee or stipulation; and that by precept, lecture, and every other mode of instruction, I will impart a knowledge of the Art to my own sons, and those of my teachers, and to disciples bound by stipulation and oath according to the law of medicine, but to none others. I will follow that system of regimen which, according to my ability and judgment I consider for the benefit of my patients, and abstain from whatever is deleterious and mischievous. I will give no deadly medicine to anyone if asked, nor suggest any such counsel; and in like manner I will not give to a woman a pessary to produce abortion. With purity and with holiness I will pass my life and practice my Art. I will not cut persons laboring under the stone, but will leave this to be done by men who are practitioners of this work. Into whatever houses I enter, I will go into them for the benefit of the sick, and will abstain from every voluntary act of mischief and corruption; and, further, from the seduction of females or males, of freeman and slaves. Whatever, in connection with my professional practice or not, in connection with it I see or hear in the life of men which ought not to be spoken of abroad, I will not divulge, as reckoning that all such should be kept secret. While I continue to keep this Oath unviolated, may it be granted to me to enjoy life and the practice of the art, respected by all men, in all times! But should I trespass and violate this Oath, may the reverse by my lot!" *(Encyclopaedia Britannica)*

Ethical Implications of the Clinical Trial System

CHAPTER NINE

Access to promising new treatments hinges on arbitrary rules enforced by the FDA. Officially, the FDA is a consumer protection agency. Most Americans believe it serves a noble purpose, especially in light of its recent publicity as the archenemy of Big Tobacco. This perception of nobility, however, is unwarranted.

The FDA has gained monopolistic control over the dispensation of medicine at virtually every level.[1] As we saw in chapter 8, the criteria it uses in its decision-making process are often arbitrary. In the following pages, we will see that the FDA enforces a clinical trial system that prevents participants from receiving optimal medical care, and sometimes denies them treatment altogether. Moreover, there are many instances where the FDA has excessively delayed treatments that have potent beneficial effects, leading to countless deaths.[2]

How can such damaging policies remain in effect? In the past, many of these policies did not matter. Experimental cancer treatments were only marginally more effective than existing treatments, and the primary concern was whether they benefited anyone at all. But now, as new treatments become increasingly effective, delays are taking an unacceptable toll. The FDA's disregard for patient welfare has created a culture of neglect in the medical community, not only affecting patients who participate in clinical trials, but jeopardizing the lives of those awaiting life-saving treatments.

Disregard for Clinical Trial Participants

Although clinical trials are needed to evaluate new treatments, they should not deprive patients of their best chance of survival. Yet clinical trials are designed to serve the interests of the larger medical community, not of the patients participating in the trials. As a result, physicians can be remarkably callous in their attitude toward clinical trial participants.

In the fall of 2000, I attended a lecture by a famous neurosurgeon, Dr. Keith Black, presented to a group of neurology residents at our local veterans hospital. Dr. Black addressed the value of surgery in increasing survival time for glioblastoma patients. He noted that controlled clinical trials had not been performed, so the issue was still disputed. One of the neurologists attending the lecture—not a resident, but a staff physician—asked why the medical community had been so slow to conduct a randomized clinical trial in which half the patients did not receive surgery. Somewhat shocked by the question, Dr. Black quickly regained his composure and replied that the absence of randomized clinical trials notwithstanding, almost all neurosurgeons were convinced that surgery did, indeed, increase survival, and to conduct such a trial would be unethical. Dissatisfied with this answer, the neurologist expressed his concern that medical science was not well served by this apparent sentimentality on the part of neurosurgeons.

In some cases, this disregard for patient welfare is institutionalized and officially sanctioned. For example, the standard protocol for phase-I clinical trials involves dose escalation to establish the safety profile and optimal dosage for a new agent. Early in the trial, patients are given very low dosages. As the trial progresses, new patients are given higher dosages until toxicity becomes evident. Even when an agent is known to be nontoxic, researchers begin with the least effective dosage.

Consider recent clinical trials with Endostatin, a drug that inhibits angiogenesis (the growth of new blood vessels, which appears essential for tumor progression). Prior to the phase-I trial, Endostatin was tested for toxicity in both rodents and monkeys; even very high dosages did not create toxic side effects. Nevertheless, early trial participants received only the lowest dosages of the treatment. Given the prior research with animal models, there was every reason to believe that these dosages would be ineffective. What purpose was served by knowingly giving terminally ill patients an ineffective dosage of a nontoxic drug? The FDA maintains that animal studies are an inadequate basis for establishing toxicity, and that something catastrophic might have occurred if the higher dosages had been used at the start. Let us grant that this was a serious, though unlikely, possibility. Given the studies already conducted, does anyone believe that the trial participants would have declined an opportunity to receive a higher dosage? Even if they were told that the higher dosage might be a serious threat to their health, their alternatives were nil. Without an effective dosage, they would be dead in a matter of months. Yet they were not permitted to risk the higher dosage, even though it was their only chance for survival. In other words, the FDA sentenced many of these patients to an almost certain death—under the guise of protecting patient interests.

The Endostatin clinical trials revealed no toxicity, even at the highest dosage. This was consistent with the data from animal studies. Of the patients who received the lowest dosages, most suffered tumor growth and presumably died. These deaths were a direct result of the FDA's lack of flexibility. Rather than allow clinical trials to build on existing scientific knowledge, the FDA forces researchers to adhere to rigid policies when conducting clinical trials. Enforcing general rules regardless of the circumstances is the forte of bureaucrats.

Disregard for Patients Awaiting Life-Saving Treatments

Flexibility is one of the major issues confronting government health policy today. Because of the biological revolution, nontoxic treatments that have a real possibility of curing cancer may soon become available. The question is, how soon? Will it take the usual five years to progress through the three-stage clinical trial process, or will dramatic results in phases I and II convince the FDA to make these treatments available more quickly? Hundreds of thousands of lives hinge on the resolution of this issue. Over 500,000 Americans die of cancer every year. Each year that we must wait for an effective treatment, we see an annual death toll that rivals American casualties in both world wars.

In a recent example, the results of a new treatment for chronic myelogenous leukemia were announced with dramatic fanfare. Known as STI-571, it is perhaps the only treatment for any form of cancer that has had a 100 percent success rate in a clinical trial. Of thirty-one patients who received the treatment in a phase-I trial, all had their white-blood-cell counts return to normal.[3] If the FDA had been concerned with patient welfare, it would have made this treatment immediately available. Yet certification did not occur even after a second trial, conducted with 550 patients, in which 90 percent of participants had their blood counts normalize. In fact, the treatment was only approved after a third clinical trial with 1,000 patients. Throughout this testing, STI-571 was shown to be less toxic than aspirin.[4]

Why were phase-III trials necessary? The point of a randomized trial is to guarantee that positive outcomes are not due to a sampling error. But it is impossible to intentionally produce a sampling bias that would result in a 100 percent success rate, much less have it occur by chance. No one could have doubted the drug's efficacy after the extraordinary phase-I results. But the FDA insisted on larger trials—at great expense to the drug developer, and at even greater cost to patients who could not participate in the clinical trials. Because these patients were denied access to a life-saving treatment, their disease worsened and many of them died. How many lives is the FDA willing to sacrifice in their adherence to contrived standards?

Ironically, the FDA congratulates itself on its expeditious certification of STI-571. When the final clinical trials were completed, it was unusually speedy in processing the application. But this does not excuse the extensive delay imposed by unnecessary additional trials.

A second example involves a biotech company named ImClone Systems Incorporated, which made the front page of the *New York Times* because of charges that its executive officers had duped shareholders. The charges were the direct result of the FDA refusing to review ImClone's application for the approval of their new product, C-225 (Erbitux). C-225 is a monoclonal antibody that targets the epidermal growth factor receptor, one of the most common cellular signaling channels to cause malignant growth. (Cancer cells commonly have many more receptors for this growth factor than normal cells, causing the cancer cells to divide wildly.) Because blocking this signaling channel usually does not kill the cancer directly, C-225 works best in combination with chemotherapy and radiation.

C-225 produced impressive results in head and neck cancer, pancreatic cancer, and advanced colon cancer. ImClone decided to seek FDA approval for C-225 as a treatment for colon cancer, based on a trial where patients who had failed chemotherapy were continued on chemotherapy in combination with the new drug. Although the FDA initially approved the design of the trial, in December 2001 it reversed its decision, contending that it could not be sure that the trial patients had failed chemotherapy before the new drug was added. Many oncologists were aghast—they had been awaiting the drug's approval and had planned to immediately begin using it with a wide variety of patients.[5] Historically, patients who fail several treatments are unlikely to benefit from additional treatment of any sort. C-225 offers hope for these patients; nevertheless, because of the FDA's action, the drug may not be available for another year.

For cancer patients, their families, and their friends, seeing a promising treatment on the horizon and knowing it will be unavailable for another one to three years is a difficult pill to swallow. An example from my own experience involves a close friend, an internationally prominent professor of psychology at Columbia University. When I learned that he had been diagnosed with small cell lung cancer, I began searching the medical literature for new treatments. Typically, the disease at first responds well to radiation and chemotherapy, then recurs within six to eighteen months, at which time the prognosis is extremely poor. My friend had responded well to the initial treatment, but options for preventing a recurrence seemed abysmal.

I discovered a phase-II study that combined a monoclonal antibody with a common bacteria to stimulate the immune system in patients with small cell lung cancer.[6] After more than four years, only 15 percent of the patients had relapsed. These results were far better than those for any other treatment previously reported. When my friend inquired about the treatment, however, he learned that the phase-II trial had been completed, and, because of exclusion criteria, he was not eligible for phase III. His ineligibility was perhaps just as well, because he did not wish to endure the 50 percent chance of being in the control group that would not receive the treatment.

Consider the implications of this situation. A treatment existed that was more promising than anything else available; without it, my friend had a high probability of a fatal recurrence within one year. In the end, FDA regulations prevented my friend from receiving this life-saving treatment, and he died.

The FDA's Approval Process Is Unnecessary

It takes many years before a new drug is made available to the public, a delay that seems especially unreasonable when we consider the difference between the initial approval process and off-label usage. When the FDA approves a drug for one indication, that drug can be prescribed for other conditions as well. Often these off-label usages have a larger impact than the original usage. Thalidomide, for example, was approved only for leprosy, but it is now used for lupus, Crohn's disease, multiple myeloma, and HIV-related diseases such as Kaposi's sarcoma. It also has shown some degree of effectiveness for several other kinds of cancer, including gliomas.

Off-label prescription is an invaluable component of medicine's arsenal of treatments. And because the FDA is not involved in their approval, off-label usages are immediately available to the public. If the medical community can be trusted to use drugs for purposes other than the original indication, why must the original indication surmount a separate, more arduous set of FDA hurdles? The financial cost of such oversight is enormous, and thousands of lives are lost before a new drug makes its way through the lengthy approval process. This could only occur because a government bureaucracy has managed to enlarge its domain of power at the expense of public interest.

But it is not only the government at fault. The mainstream medical establishment is equally to blame because it has done everything in its power to differentiate itself from alternative medicine. Modern medicine does not want to be considered a healing art. It wants to be a science. So it has rushed to adopt a set of inappropriate criteria as a basis for accepting or excluding new treatments. These criteria were borrowed from other scientific disciplines that have very different questions at issue. At the same time, the concerns truly relevant to medicine have been ignored. In the process of erecting this barrier of "scientific evaluation," mainstream medicine has become insensitive to its real purpose: to provide each patient with the best medical care available.

It is true that many promising new treatments, like that for small cell lung cancer, have uncertainties that need to be resolved. But most terminally ill patients would rather risk uncertainty than settle for traditional options. And most oncologists, if diagnosed with a terminal illness, would do everything in their power to obtain these new treatments. Yet they seem so hamstrung by the rules of their profession that they are quite willing to deny these treatments to their own patients.

Physicians who conduct clinical trials naively assume that a statistically significant difference between a treatment and control group allows a meaningful inference about an agent's potential benefits. But there are precious few cancer patients who care if the treatment they are considering had a statistically significant effect when presented to a randomly assigned group of 500 patients relative to a comparable group of patients who do not receive the treatment. Each cancer patient is concerned about his or her own welfare. Unless the clinical trial allows patients to make meaningful judgments about a treatment's likely benefit, the difference between the treatment and control groups does not matter one iota.

ENDNOTES

1. The original authority of the FDA, provided by the Food, Drug and Cosmetic Act of 1938, was limited to regulating safety. Companies seeking to market a new drug had to submit a New Drug Application citing evidence that the drug was safe to use. In 1962, in the aftermath of the thalidomide tragedy in Europe, Senator Carey Estes Kefauver amended this act, allowing the FDA to set the standards for determining a drug's efficacy. Since the thalidomide issue related to safety and not efficacy, what was the rationale for Kefauver's amendment? While there is no definitive answer to this question, the reason stated at the time was to reduce the costs incurred by consumers for ineffective drugs. That is, the bill assumed that the consumer and the medical community were too dumb to know whether a drug was doing any good, so the

FDA was assigned the task of making that decision for them. Since then, the FDA's power has grown, and it now attempts to regulate even what a drug manufacturer says about its drugs. For example, aspirin manufacturers may not advertise their product as a preventive agent for heart attacks, even though this effect has been well documented and a daily baby aspirin is a frequent medical recommendation.

2.   Gieringer, D. H. Compassion vs. control: FDA investigational drug regulation. *Cato Institute Policy Analysis.* 1986 May 20;72. Also see Goldberg, R. Food and Drug Administration. In: Boaz, D., and Crane, E. H., eds. *The Cato Handbook for Congress.* Washington, D.C.: Cato Institute; 1995.

3.   Leukemia drug heralds molecularly targeted era. *Journal of the National Cancer Institute.* 2000;92(1):6-8.

4.   New pill touted as "holy grail" of leukemia research. *The Houston Chronicle.* 2000 Nov 2.

5.   Oncologists were not alone in their concern that a promising new treatment would not become available. Even the conservative *Wall Street Journal* (2002 Feb 13) criticized the FDA for delaying its review of a new drug in "Bullying ImClone: What Does the FDA Have Against Saving Lives?"

6.   Grant, S. C., et al. Long survival of patients with small-cell lung cancer after adjuvant treatment with the anti-idiotypic antibody BEC2 plus *Bacillus Calmette-Gúerin. Clinical Cancer Research.* 1999;5(6):1319-1323.

Phase-III Trials: Gold Standard or Fool's Gold?

CHAPTER TEN

A PEDESTRIAN ENCOUNTERS A DRUNK MAN ON HIS HANDS AND KNEES near an intersection. "What are you doing?" the pedestrian asks.

"Looking for my house key," the drunk man replies.

"Where did you lose it?"

"About ten feet up the sidewalk."

"Then why are you looking here?"

"This is where the light is."

This well-known story provides a meaningful analogy to what is now official government policy for evaluating new cancer treatments. Rather than judge a new treatment on the magnitude of its clinical benefits, the FDA relies on a method of evaluation drawn from the basic sciences, where the purpose of analysis is radically different. This method, used in phase-III clinical trials, focuses on whether an agent produces a statistically significant difference between a treatment group and a control group.

Methods for conducting clinical trials must be evaluated in terms of how well they advance clinical knowledge. For brain tumors and other fatal diseases, the clinical trial system has been an abysmal failure. To date, none of the information produced by clinical trials will help brain tumor patients make basic life-and-death decisions, including:

- Should I go immediately from radiation to chemotherapy, or delay chemotherapy until my tumor recurs?
- Given my profile (age, tumor size, and so forth), will additional radiation, such as radiosurgery or brachytherapy, improve my survival time?
- Does chemotherapy generally improve survival? If so, how much? Enough to justify the decrease in my quality of life?
- Does chemotherapy work for some people but not others (such as younger patients vs. older patients)?

Any set of testing procedures that has not answered such basic questions can hardly be commended for its efficiency. Moreover, it should not be relied on to determine which treatments a patient is allowed to receive outside of clinical trials.

If the FDA's mission is to protect the public, it should not be in the business of preventing patients from receiving new, potentially life-saving treatments. On the contrary, it should facilitate access to new treatments as rapidly as possible. To do this, two things must change:

1) For diseases that currently have no effective treatment, the FDA and the medical community must abandon the requirement of phase-III clinical trials.

2) Physicians conducting clinical trials must report data for individual trial participants in order to identify a treatment's effects in specific subpopulations. Only then can we predict the likelihood that a treatment will benefit a given patient.

Why Abandon Phase-III Trials?

The expense of phase-III clinical trials is a driving force behind the high cost of newly developed drugs, which so often arouses the ire of politicians and the public. More importantly, throughout the typical two to four years required to complete phase-III trials, many lives are needlessly lost while patients await approval for treatments that have already demonstrated efficacy in phase II.

Equally disturbing is the fact that many promising agents never find their way to phase-III trials, and when they do, flawed statistical procedures often obscure the treatments' true effects, thereby preventing FDA certification. The notion that new treatments must show a .05 level of statistical significance in a random-assignment clinical trial is simply unacceptable, especially when we consider the misguided methodology on which this evaluation is based.

THE NULL HYPOTHESIS

At the end of a phase-III trial, clinicians compare the outcome for patients in the treatment group to that of patients in the control group. This difference is analyzed using "null hypothesis testing," a statistical method borrowed from the social sciences. This method was created for a nonmedical purpose, and it is fundamentally inappropriate for advancing medical care. In fact, it imposes an enormous conservative bias in identifying effective treatments.

Null hypothesis testing begins with the assumption (the null hypothesis) that any difference between the treatment and control groups could be due to variability in the patients' characteristics (such as age or treatment history), not to the experimental agent. Researchers must disprove this assumption before the treatment will be regarded as effective. To do this, they must demonstrate that the difference between the treatment and control groups is statistically significant—that there is a low probability (less than .05) that the difference is due to factors other than the treatment.

In my own field of experimental psychology, null hypothesis testing is generally regarded as an acceptable statistical approach. And, as a reviewer for numerous psychology journals, I have had many occasions to evaluate whether the statistical procedures used in individual experiments are appropriate for their purpose. In such experiments, null hypothesis testing is used to establish the validity of a hypothesis of a general nature. We choose rigid statistical criteria (such as probability values of .05 or .01) because we do not want our general scientific principles to be subject to doubt.

The purpose of medical research, however, is not to establish general scientific principles, but to identify treatments that are likely to have some clinical benefit. Rigid statistical criteria are inappropriate here because they create "false negatives," increasing the risk that a promising new treatment will be rejected.

Although null hypothesis testing is widely used in several scientific disciplines, it seems that its conceptual foundation is not well understood by medical researchers. The failure to find a statistically significant difference routinely leads researchers to conclude that a treatment is ineffective, but the logic of null hypothesis testing does not, in fact, permit this inference. All the failure allows is the conclusion that a statistically significant effect has not yet been demonstrated. Acceptance of the null hypothesis is a common conceptual error in the medical community. Absence of evidence is not evidence of absence: just because a clinical trial failed to detect a statistically significant difference does not mean that another trial using a better methodology would do the same.

STATISTICAL NOISE
Statistical significance depends on the size of the difference between the treatment and the control group compared to the overall variability in outcome among patients in the control group. If the patient population is extremely heterogeneous, the benefits of a treatment may be obscured. Identifying the true effects of the treatment becomes a signal

detection problem, much like that confronted by engineers who must separate a coherent signal from background noise. But in clinical trials, the methods used to extract this signal are primitive.

In the ideal world, subjects in the treatment group would be identical to those in the control group in every respect, except one group would receive the treatment and the other would not. In reality, patients differ along many dimensions, some of which help determine clinical outcome. For brain tumor trials, three factors are known to be of major importance: age, Karnofsky score, and treatment history. These factors often play a greater role in patient outcome than whether or not that patient receives an experimental treatment. Therefore, when a treatment agent is tested in a clinical trial, it is important to ensure that the effects of the treatment are not swamped by the effects of patient characteristics. This statistical noise can be factored out, allowing the effects of the treatment to be seen more clearly.[1] But as odd as it may seem, the evaluation procedure sanctioned by the FDA does not attempt to control this statistical noise. As a result, many agents are judged as ineffective even though more powerful procedures would show them to be effective.[2]

Clinicians understand that age, Karnofsky score, treatment history, and other factors can play an important role in determining the outcome of a clinical trial. This is why they randomly assign patients to either a treatment group or control group. They assume that the effects of extraneous factors will be canceled out when they are represented equally in the two arms of the experimental design. In principle, this is true; however, if many factors contribute to the statistical noise, they may produce so much variability that a statistically significant effect still will not be detected. Therefore, it is critically important to recognize that phase-III trial results may say more about the variability among trial participants than about the efficacy of an experimental treatment.

As an example, suppose a clinical trial involved twelve pairs of identical twins, with one member of each pair receiving the experimental treatment while the other received the control condition. In each case, the twin receiving the experimental treatment had a better clinical outcome. Clearly the treatment was effective. But suppose the same twenty-four patients were randomly assigned to a treatment or control group. If the different sets of twins varied widely in age, the trial most likely would fail to produce a statistically significant difference. The treatment would be regarded as ineffective and consequently rejected for clinical use.

Treatment benefits frequently go undetected in phase-III clinical trials. Given that these trials are potentially misleading, it is foolhardy to ignore treatments that showed promising results in phase II simply because they did not meet the strict standards required in phase III.

MISGUIDED GOALS

Oncology's too eager rejection of treatments that have failed phase III is only part of the problem. Far more serious is the goal underlying the current strategy for evaluating new treatments: to identify agents that produce a statistically significant improvement in the mean or median outcome when patients receiving a treatment are compared to an equivalent set of patients not receiving the treatment.

If a trial produces a median survival time that is three months longer for the treatment group than for the control group, and the difference is statistically significant, what does this tell the patient? Does it mean that the patient will live three months longer if he or she receives the treatment? Certainly not.

First, there is extensive overlap in patient outcome. Any patient in the control group might do better than any given patient in the treatment group, and vice versa. Second, because clinical trials require a large number of patients, treatments need only produce minimal benefits to show a statistically significant effect.[3] This is the nature of statistical analysis. When large samples are used, even small differences in outcome will be judged as statistically significant, while smaller samples will fail to yield a significant difference unless the effect of the treatment is quite large.

Whether the difference in median survival time is statistically significant offers information only at the grossest level. It will not predict the likelihood of a beneficial effect, much less the size of the effect, for any given patient. In the real world, treatment outcomes are probabilistic. A treatment that helps one patient may not help, or may even harm, another. Both patients and physicians need to know the probability of these different outcomes.[4]

Currently, the aim of clinical trials is to determine whether one treatment is better than another (or better than a placebo). A more appropriate goal would be to estimate the likelihood that a treatment will benefit a given patient. This can only be accomplished by relating the individual characteristics of trial participants to the effects of the experimental treatment. Because phase-III trials focus on statistical significance, they typically ignore the effects of individual differences on treatment outcome.

When I first began reading the clinical trials literature, I was surprised and dismayed to find that the majority of trial results excluded information that was most essential to patients. Given the amount of effort and expense involved in conducting a clinical trial, it is astonishing how little information is typically extracted from the results. The most egregious examples are trials that report only median survival times, along with a statistical assessment of whether the differences are reliable. For example, glioblastoma clinical trials show that chemotherapy produces a median survival time of eleven to twelve months. They do not report the percentage of patients that will benefit from the treatment. While chemotherapy will provide a significant improvement for a minority of patients, the critical information is how many patients are helped and what type of patients are most likely to receive the benefit.

Developing Patient Profiles

Cancer treatments are not benign procedures, and patients must make a cost-benefit analysis to determine which treatments might be worthwhile to endure. Rather than look at median outcomes from phase-III clinical trials, patients need to see outcomes for trial participants who are most like themselves. Individual differences matter, and patients are more likely to predict a treatment's benefit if they see how it affected patients who share their specific profile. For this reason, it is essential that clinical trials report individual subject data.

Many phase-II trials already publish results for every trial participant, as well as data about age, tumor grade, and other characteristics. This information enables patients to identify clinical trial participants who are most like themselves. Based on the outcomes of specific trial participants, individual patients can make an educated guess about what kind of effect the treatment would have on them.

To make such an assessment, the clinical outcome of patients receiving a new treatment must be compared to "historical controls," similar patients from years past who did not receive the treatment.[5] We can determine if an experimental treatment will increase survival time for a specific patient profile—for example, brain tumor patients over sixty years of age who have a Karnofsky score of 90—by comparing their average outcome to that of corresponding historical controls. If the experimental treatment improves clinical outcome for each patient category, this would indicate that the treatment is generally effective. If there are large differences in outcome among the different patient profiles, the treatment should be restricted to those categories for which it exceeded the historical controls.

The database of historical controls needs to be large enough to establish reliable baselines of clinical outcome for different patient profiles. The more historical controls, the greater the number of possible patient categories. Thus, an essential step to improving clinical outcome is to develop a large, Internet-accessible database, where raw data for individual patients is recorded at the end of every clinical trial. Even if those who conduct the trials have no interest in developing the detailed information, archiving the data would allow other investigators to analyze the results. Such archives would greatly increase the number of patients with well-defined profiles, improving our ability to predict the effectiveness of a treatment for specific individuals. The National Cancer Institute or another prominent cancer organization would be responsible for maintaining the archives.

Using patient profiles and historical controls would negate the primary concern that motivates the FDA, and clinical researchers generally, to require randomized phase-III trials: the difficulty in knowing whether trial participants are representative of the larger patient population. For example, participants in a given trial might be much younger than the average patient. If patients in a phase-II trial are partitioned according to age and other criteria that are known to determine clinical outcome, each category could then be compared to its own historical control. This would reduce the concern that the subjects in a given trial are unrepresentative.

The Benefits of Phase-II Trials

By glorifying phase-III clinical trials, we ignore evidence from phase-II trials even when it suggests that a new treatment has a high probability of success. For example, a phase-II trial testing Poly-ICLC with anaplastic astrocytoma patients produced a median stabilization period of 5.4 years, with ten of eleven patients still alive at the time the study was reported.[6] When I described these results to my neuro-oncologist, he dismissed the findings as impossible and implied that something must have been wrong with the study. In fact, the trial was subsequently published in one of the major science journals, and I found it to be of unusually high quality in its detailed description of both the procedures and results. Yet, for whatever reason, it has not advanced to phase-III trials and presumably may never do so. As a result, the treatment is generally unavailable. When the results are compared to historical controls, however, there is no question that Poly-ICLC represents a major advance in the treatment of anaplastic astrocytoma. If we abandoned phase-III trials, Poly-ICLC would be widely used today.

The elimination of phase-III trials would reduce the cost of healthcare and save countless lives, not only by increasing the chances of identifying beneficial treatments, but also by making these treatments immediately available to the public. Moreover, the use of historical controls, rather than the current phase-III procedure of randomly assigning half the subjects to the control condition, would discourage the use of placebo controls. Two recent glioblastoma trials, involving Gliadel and marimastat, used placebos, claiming that there were no beneficial treatments available. This is one of the most extreme cases of accepting the null hypothesis that I have seen. If it were actually true, then there would be no rationale for giving any treatment to a brain tumor patient. This, of course, is not the case. Current clinical practice is predicated on the assumption that some glioblastoma patients will benefit from the traditional treatments. There is no justification for abandoning that assumption in clinical trials. Moreover, if patients in the control group believe that they may be receiving the experimental treatment, they will be discouraged from pursuing alternative treatments that may be beneficial (such as tamoxifen).

The best way to predict a treatment's effect on a given patient is to look at the effects it produced in similar patients. Oncologists who conduct clinical trials will probably regard this as a retreat from the scientific rigor of phase-III trials, which provides an explicit set of rules for evaluating new treatments. There is no question that the method I advocate depends on intuitive judgment. But this shortcoming must be balanced against the fact that random-assignment phase-III clinical trials often produce erroneous information.

Consider early clinical trials on the effects of chemotherapy for brain tumor patients. At the time, it was customary not to distinguish between patients with glioblastomas and those with anaplastic astrocytomas. Both tumors were treated as "high-grade gliomas" and were expected to have a similar response to treatment. (We now know that different grades of tumors have different prognoses, primarily because grade-III tumors respond better to radiation and chemotherapy.) The results of these trials were quite inconsistent; some showed that chemotherapy had a statistically significant effect and some did not. Eventually a consensus emerged that chemotherapy did, indeed, produce a statistically significant benefit, and it became the standard of care in the United States.

In retrospect, the inconsistent results were due to the mixing of diagnostic categories. But the important lesson is that the information provided by those clinical trials was misleading for both categories. It underestimated the benefit of chemotherapy for the lower-grade tumors, and it overestimated the benefit for glioblastoma patients. In what way did these randomized phase-III trials—the gold standard of evidence—advance clinical knowledge about which treatments will be effective for different categories of patients?

If the researchers had reported the entire distribution of outcomes along with individual subject data (including tumor type), it would have been clear that chemotherapy had a different effect on different tumors. It is important to appreciate the generality of this issue. If it is a mistake to mix results for different diagnoses, then it is also a mistake to mix results for different ages, Karnofsky scores, treatment histories, and so forth.

Individual characteristics may be the dominant variables in determining whether treatments are effective, and it is only a matter of time before patient profiles assume a critical role in evaluating new agents. In fact, advances in genetics research indicate that genetic typology is related to treatment outcome. A recent study involving a gene that repairs DNA damage found that glioblastoma patients who have a defective gene more often respond to chemotherapy (BCNU) than patients who do not have a defective gene.[7] Presumably, the intact gene quickly repairs damage caused by chemotherapy, making malignant cells more resistant to the cytotoxic effects of the treatment. This gene appears to mediate chemotherapy resistance for many other malignant tumors as well. There is no doubt that clinical trials of the future will take such important genetic differences into consideration. But today, there is no excuse for ignoring known differences like age and Karnofsky score.

The goal of oncology is to provide treatments that offer the best possible chance for survival. If a new treatment shows promising results in phase-II, that treatment should be made immediately available. This would restrict the FDA to assessing treatment toxicity (overseeing phase-I trials) and monitoring clinical results reported by physicians using the drug. If results are inconsistent with those demonstrated in phase-II trials, only then should the FDA determine if a drug is ineffective and should be removed from the market.

Current procedures for evaluating new treatments are not in the best interests of cancer patients. This is not intended to be a blanket indictment of the importance of phase-III clinical trials.[8] But for diseases that have no effective treatment, phase-III trials impose long delays and an illegitimate filtering of treatment options that result in many deaths. Any agency that has a mission to protect the public should not be in the business of thwarting patients from receiving new treatments that might save their lives. I can think of no other arena in which the most basic human rights have been so trampled, and with such awful consequences.

ENDNOTES

1. In psychology and other social sciences, the primary statistical procedure for isolating different sources of variance is called Analysis of Variance. This procedure separates the effects due to variables (and their interactions) that are part of the experimental design from the remaining variance, known as noise or "error variance." If this statistical procedure were applied to clinical trials, the analysis would isolate not only the effects of the treatment, but also the effects of age and Karnofsky score. Analysis of Variance reduces the error variance because it extracts effects that can be ascribed to identifiable variables. Detecting the true effect of an experimental treatment is much easier when there is a small amount of error variance.

2. Most cancer clinical trials report several statistical analyses. The preferred approach has been to analyze the differences between survival curves for the treatment and control groups. The standard test is a variation of a chi-square, which calculates the probability that the proportion of survivors for given time epochs is disproportionately in favor of the treatment condition. The reason for this approach is that many subjects are lost before a clinical trial is completed, and researchers want to keep as much of their data as possible. Unfortunately, the analysis ignores the possibility that a treatment may show a different effect later in the trial. For example, in glioblastoma trials comparing radiation vs. a combination of radiation and chemotherapy, the standard analysis failed to reveal a statistically significant difference. However, given that chemotherapy increases the average two-year survival rate by a factor of 3 to 6, this conclusion is misleading. Any test that does not validate such a large difference has fundamental shortcomings.

The second type of clinical trial analysis, called Cox Proportional Hazards Analysis, isolates the effects of individual variables (such as age) by statistically holding constant the values of all the other variables. This method extracts what would otherwise be statistical noise so the effect of the experimental treatment can be more easily seen. As far as I have been able to determine, the FDA does not utilize the results from Cox Proportional Hazards Analysis. This is unfortunate, because the survival time analysis, which is of primary importance in FDA decisions, allows extraneous factors to undercut scientific assessment of the treatment's true effects. Why not take age, Karnofsky score, and other variables out of the equation, since the issue in question is whether the treatment is efficacious? The Cox Proportional Hazard model does not identify interactions between such variables. Analysis of Variance, described in note 1 above, does.

The third type of statistical analysis, seen in recent clinical trials, is called Multiple Regression. In principle, this model isolates not only the effects of age, Karnofsky score, sex, and other variables, but also the interactions between them. However, Multiple Regression Analysis assumes that each variable is normally distributed. This is rarely the case, which largely undermines the validity of the multiple regression probability values as an indicator of the odds that any treatment effect is not due to chance. Analysis of Variance depends on similar assumptions; however, computer simulations show that violations of these assumptions only affect the validity of this model in rare cases. Analysis of Variance depends on the central limit theorem, which converts any distribution of the original population of scores into a normal distribution of sample statistics. Multiple Regression, on the other hand, does not utilize the correcting effects of the central limit theorem.

3. There is a critical statistical distinction between "effect size" and level of statistical significance. Effect size is the percentage of the total variance in the results that can be ascribed to the experimental variable. When the number of subjects is increased, the effect size stays constant, whereas the required level of significance is easier to achieve. The effect size is of greater importance.

4. There are statistical methods, known as "dominance statistics," that provide a straightforward estimate of the likelihood that a treatment will benefit an individual patient. An example is a variation of one of the most commonly used nonparametric statistics, the Mann-Whitney U. When the U value is divided by the product of the sample sizes of the treatment and control groups, the result is an exact probability that a randomly drawn subject from the treatment group exceeds in outcome a randomly drawn subject from the control group. This statistic would be preferable to that currently used by the FDA, because it addresses the issue most important to patients—the likelihood that a treatment will be effective. Unfortunately, like all nonparametric statistics, this approach does not extract variance due to other factors, nor does it identify variance due to interactions between the experimental treatment and individual differences (such as age).

5. Several neuro-oncology centers, including M.D. Anderson in Houston, have begun to use historical controls rather than devote extensive time and resources to phase-III trials. They use a database that categorizes glioma patients according to age, tumor grade, and other variables, resulting in six classes of patients. These different classes have survival times that vary by a multiple of 10. To test the results of an experimental treatment, researchers compare the outcome of individual patients who received the treat-

ment to patients in corresponding categories within the database. Such comparisons have sometimes contradicted results produced in phase-III clinical trials. For example, brachytherapy was shown to be ineffective in at least one large-scale phase-III trial, and many investigators have argued that benefits reported in phase-II trials were due to a selection bias. However, when patients who received the treatment were categorized and compared to historical controls, brachytherapy was shown to increase survival rates for each of the six categories of patients, with the largest improvement occurring in patients with the worst prognosis. (Videtic, G. M., et al. Use of the RTOG recursive partitioning analysis to validate the benefit of iodine-125 implants in the primary treatment of malignant gliomas. *International Journal of Radiation Oncology, Biology, Physics.* 1999;45[2]:687-692.)

6. See chapter 2, note 6.

7. Esteller, M., et al. Inactivation of the DNA-repair gene MGMT and the clinical response of gliomas to alkylating agents. *New England Journal of Medicine.* 2000;343(19):1408-1409.

8. There are situations in which phase-III trials are useful and informative. If a disease has an effective treatment, new treatments should be tested against it in a phase-III trial. Even in such circumstances, however, it is important to recognize that the test would be much more powerful if it went beyond randomization to include partitioning of subjects according to individual differences that are known to affect clinical outcome.

Bastille Day for Cancer Patients

For patients with deadly diagnoses, medical practice and government policy must be revised. We need greater flexibility in exploring new treatment options, as well as immediate access to promising treatments that have not yet passed the scrutiny of current FDA regulatory policies. We must ensure that patients receive optimal care during clinical trials, and that clinicians report patient profiles and clinical results for all trial participants. Most of all, we need greater flexibility and imagination in developing new treatment approaches beyond the "one size fits all" mentality that dominates medical thinking.

I have developed relationships with scores of brain tumor patients over the past three to four years. Most of these people have died from their disease. Most received no assistance in developing a treatment program beyond what was originally prescribed. A few succeeded in persuading their oncologist to prescribe tamoxifen, but none of them convinced their oncologist to cooperate with a combinational treatment, even though several physicians agreed that it seemed like a good idea. Although the efficacy of both Accutane and thalidomide are sup-ported by credible evidence from phase-II trials, most oncologists have been unwilling to add them to their treatment protocols.

Few physicians appreciate the value of treatments developed outside of mainstream American oncology, including melatonin, mushroom extracts such as PSK, and polyunsaturated fatty acids such as gamma-linolenic acid. Part of this is simply ignorance, but a more fundamental problem is that these treatments have not been officially sanctioned. Without that sanction, neither the clinical literature in other countries nor the nontoxic nature of these treatments is relevant.

Being an oncologist is not an easy job. Dealing with dying, desper-ate, and often miserable people is extraordinarily demanding. The task becomes yet more difficult when patients have unrealistic expectations about magic "cures" that are sometimes championed by those outside of conventional medicine. It is easy to sympathize with oncology's need for rigid standards of evidence to provide a bulwark against such claims. But it is not easy to accept the irrational manner in which this bulwark has been constructed.

The logic of clinical trials is fundamentally faulty, and it has cost thousands of lives. By requiring phase-III clinical trials, we not only lengthen the time before effective treatments become available, we pre-vent treatments with known efficacy from reaching consumers. Many agents will never advance to phase-III trials simply because they lack adequate sponsorship to prevail against FDA regulatory policies. This was true for Accutane, tamoxifen, and most of the other components of my treatment program. But it is especially troublesome for treatments extensively evaluated and accepted without question in other countries.

Fighting for Our Lives

Cancer patients do not have to accept this. We have a model for deal-ing with many of these problems: the gay community and its fight to develop a treatment for AIDS. The gay community established its own knowledge base about treatment alternatives, and this knowledge was quickly and widely disseminated. When new treatments appeared on the horizon, the community fought to make them immediately available, bypassing the clinical trial process that would have delayed availability for three to five years. The AIDS cocktail, responsible for saving, or at least prolonging, the lives of many thousands of people, was never subjected to phase-III clinical trials. Government officials simply could not withstand the political heat. If the FDA had prevailed in its attempts to require the usual evaluation procedure, consider what the cost would have been. Cancer patients are still paying that cost.

Hopefully, the Internet will provoke similar activism among cancer patients who, up until now, have been remarkably uncritical of the government's oversight of new treatment development. The cancer community is so diffuse that no organizing body has emerged to spearhead its interests. Moreover, lobbying efforts have not been supported by the major nongovernmental cancer organizations, such as the American Cancer Society, which often act like cheerleading squads for the policies of conventional medicine.

It is difficult to predict when enough political pressure will coalesce to produce changes in current medical regulatory policies. In the interim, cancer patients no longer have to accept their oncologists' decisions about treatment. Communication technology makes knowledge more accessible, and cancer patients can use this knowledge to question their oncologists' judgment. As patients demand to know why other treatment options are not acceptable possibilities, oncologists will need to become more knowledgeable—and more flexible—about options that lie outside the medical guild's officially recommended treatments.

Better Options for Cancer Patients

At the beginning of this book, I noted that medicine is not an exact science but a probabilistic enterprise in which the outcome of virtually every cancer treatment is uncertain. Treatments that benefit a minority of patients produce no benefit, and usually considerable hardship, for the majority. This fact is central to the theme of this book. Even if the best available treatments had a 50 percent chance of benefiting a given patient, we still would need more flexible procedures for certifying new treatments. Rather than evaluate individual treatments in a piecemeal fashion, we should consider treatment cocktails—especially when agents are relatively nontoxic—a frontline possibility.

Consider an example from my own experience, which I described in an earlier chapter. After I was diagnosed with a glioblastoma, my neuro-oncologist told me that I would be dead within eighteen months, if I were lucky. Yet when I informed him that I wanted to take tamoxifen in combination with the chemotherapy he had prescribed, he was concerned about the potential danger. I had no basis for evaluating the risk, other than a brief telephone conversation with a nurse involved in a stage-II clinical trial that combined tamoxifen with BCNU. She informed me that the tamoxifen created no additional toxicity, except for an increased risk of blood clots, and that the combination seemed to increase survival rates for glioblastoma patients. This information was confirmed a couple years later when the results of the clinical trial were reported at a national cancer meeting.[1] The median survival time for glioblastoma patients receiving BCNU plus tamoxifen was sixty-six weeks, somewhat but not hugely superior to the median survival time historically reported for BCNU alone (fifty to sixty weeks). But much more important were the survival rates after two years (45 percent) and after three years (24 percent). Simply adding tamoxifen to the standard glioblastoma treatment produced a dramatic improvement in patient outcome. Because only twenty-three patients were involved in the trial, we do not know how reliable the results were. But, given that a significant proportion of glioblastoma patients receive BCNU by itself, and that tamoxifen adds little toxicity to the treatment, why should patients not add tamoxifen to the usual treatment regimen? Yet they are not informed of this possibility, and when they discover it on their own they are discouraged from pursuing it.

Once we acknowledge the probabilistic nature of cancer treatment, it becomes evident that the most rationale treatment strategy is to combine as many treatment modalities as possible, taking into consideration availability and toxicity. In earlier chapters I discussed conventional drugs such as tamoxifen, Accutane, and thalidomide, as well as essential fatty acids and mushroom extracts. The following chapters will describe many of these, as well as other potentially effective treatments, in greater detail. Some of these agents can be combined with little or no toxicity.

I believe it is possible to develop an effective combination of treatments now, rather than wait for the medical establishment to sanction a cocktail treatment. Most oncologists fail to entertain the possibility that a multipronged approach to treatment may be superior to the conventional, one-approved-drug-at-a-time approach. This reflects a lack of imagination that can be understood only in terms of professional indoctrination. It also ignores the fact that the conventional approach has been an abysmal failure.

Informed, intelligent patients who have a fatal diagnosis will not be bound by medical conventions—even if it means they must be aggressive in dealing with their oncologists, however difficult this may be. The simple fact is, these patients will die if their treatment is confined to their oncologists' recommendations. Physicians control treatment availability, but only to an extent. Many potentially effective treatments do not require prescriptions, and those that do often can be obtained over the Internet. Furthermore, patients can seek out the few oncologists who are flexible enough to see beyond their allegiance to a misunderstood Hippocratic oath.

The critical reader will recognize that what I am advocating comes perilously close to alternative medicine. In the past five years, I have become more sympathetic to alternative medicine, or at least to the component better described as "complementary medicine." Its practitioners expend considerable effort identifying naturally occurring, relatively nontoxic substances that have a credible basis for providing a treatment benefit. They have been quick to see the value in combining drugs that have only a small effect individually, but a large effect when taken together. Though alternative treatments are ignored by conventional medicine, many have shown considerable efficacy, and it is only a matter of time before these are accepted as standard medical practice.

Despite the obstacles imposed by the FDA and the medical community, there are grounds for optimism. Scientific advances will soon make today's standard cancer treatments relics of the past, not unlike frontal lobotomies used for schizophrenia. The biological revolution is producing dramatic successes at an accelerating rate. My hope is that these developments will come sooner rather than later, and that the regulatory powers will facilitate, rather than thwart, their early availability. Thousands of lives hang in the balance.

ENDNOTES

1. See chapter 8, note 8.

What Your Oncologist Won't Tell You

SECTION THREE

CANCER PATIENTS SHORTCHANGE THEMSELVES IF THEY RESTRICT their treatment options to those recommended by their oncologists. If patients take an activist approach, they can do many things to improve their chances of survival.

The following chapters advocate a number of cancer treatments, some of which are controversial. Patients are encouraged to use this information as a starting point in their own research, and to inform their physicians before using any new treatment.

Alternative Medicine

WHEN I BEGAN RESEARCHING TREATMENT OPTIONS FOR MY BRAIN tumor, I shared conventional medicine's bias against alternative medicine. As a psychologist, I knew that human beings could be gullible under the best of circumstances, much less when their health is threatened. And as someone who lived in southern California in the 1970s, I had seen myriad hucksters champion alternative lifestyles based on variations of Aquarius-age spiritualism, which I regarded as antithetical to science. In fact, my own field of psychology has had more than its share of theoretical mumbo jumbo, some of which has evolved into full-fledged disciplines though supported by only the flimsiest evidence. (Freudian psychoanalytic theory is a prime example. Ironically, conventional medicine takes Freudian theory quite seriously; it is routinely taught in most medical schools.) To my mind, alternative medicine occupied a similar niche within conventional medicine.

My negative view was not based on any serious study of alternative treatments; rather, it reflected a common derision toward "quack cures" that supposedly have been discredited. I also knew that some varieties of alternative medicine (such as homeopathy and anthroposophy) originated from ideas best described as quasi-occult. But patients with terminal cancer cannot afford to leave any stone unturned. I therefore decided to learn enough about alternative medicine to determine if it offered anything more promising than conventional medicine.

I bought a book entitled *Alternative Medicine Definitive Guide to Cancer*, by Diamond, Cowden, and Goldberg.[1] It describes a collection of cancer treatment plans and individual success stories from twenty-three alternative practitioners. The majority of these are MDs who received additional training in some variety of alternative medicine or who adapted their clinical practice to incorporate nonconventional treatments. The remaining contributors are trained naturopaths and chiropractors.

The book describes nutritional and botanical supplements, methods for enhancing the immune system, and chemical compounds eschewed by the mainstream. It also includes a lengthy discussion about the politics of cancer treatment and why patients should distrust the assertion that alternative medicine has no value. Overall, the book provides a broad introduction to alternative treatments and philosophies, showing the heterogeneity of this amorphous category of medicine.

While individual practitioners of alternative medicine differ in their specific recommendations, they share the philosophy that each individual presents a unique medical profile that must be addressed on its own terms. Thus, when two patients have the same diagnosis, their treatments may differ. A holistic approach makes it difficult to know why a specific treatment combination might be effective. This lack of scientific analysis seems not to pose a problem for advocates of alternative medicine, because they believe that medicine should be an art rather than a science. To them, a good physician is one who can examine a patient and tailor an effective treatment for that individual. It should come as no surprise, then, that the evidence supporting this approach comes not from statistical analysis but from a collection of success stories.[2]

The more I learned about alternative medicine, the more critical I became of practitioners' failure to document the efficacy of their treatments.[3] Anecdotal evidence is of little value in determining whether to take a treatment seriously, though it might provide the foundation of further investigation. At the same time I became increasingly interested in the idea that combinational treatments, especially those that boost the immune system, may be an improvement over the individual treatments offered by conventional medicine. I also noted that many of the supplements I was taking based on my own independent research were used in holistic treatment packages. Given that these had been ignored by conventional medicine in spite of persuasive evidence, I was reluctant to dismiss other alternative treatments without further investigation.

What Is Alternative Medicine?

Surveys report that 40 to 70 percent of cancer patients use some form of alternative medicine. Of these, less than half inform their oncologists. Despite its prevalence, alternative medicine is damned by the majority of American oncologists, though more and more adopt a "don't ask, don't tell" attitude with their patients.

Alternative treatments include a wide range of therapies, supplements, and lifestyle changes. Certain diets, for example, are believed to remove various toxic agents that enhance carcinogenesis. Other detoxification therapies include enemas, the removal of silver fillings in teeth, avoidance of fluorinated and chlorinated water, and chelation (a procedure by which heavy metals, toxins, and metabolic waste products are supposedly extracted from body tissue by binding with a chemical known as EDTA).

The most common alternative treatments include minerals, vitamins, and herbs, often in large dosages. Proponents believe that such supplements enhance the immune system and, in some cases, have direct anticancer effects. Meditation and visual imaging are also common, as these are said to decrease the debilitating effects of stress.[4]

Patients with serious illness use alternative medicine in one of three ways. Many take vitamins, alter their diet, and make other lifestyle changes to supplement conventional treatments. Some explore alternative treatments after the standard treatments have failed. Still others use alternative therapies in place of conventional medicine because they believe that standard treatments do more harm than good.

The widespread use of alternative medicine has been either ignored or actively opposed by conventional practitioners. Even when recommended treatments have failed and alternative medicine is the only option, many oncologists discourage its use, arguing that it creates false hope and may deplete financial resources. But oncologists are far more adamant in their opposition when patients seek to replace conventional medicine altogether.

The Chemotherapy Controversy

If a patient decides to forgo conventional treatment, it is not unreasonable to seek other treatments—even unproven treatments—that might provide benefits without causing severe side effects. One of my colleagues at the University of California made such a decision. Diagnosed with metastatic prostate cancer at age forty-nine, he switched to a macrobiotic diet. It has been fourteen years, and he has only now resorted to androgen-suppressive drugs to control his disease.

The characterization of standard cancer treatment as "slash, burn, and poison" is not unfounded, and many patients endure a great deal of misery with little benefit. Undoubtedly, lives have been shortened by conventional treatment, but that is the risk we take when we undergo some of the most severe treatments that medicine has devised. Whether it is rational to accept this risk depends on the treatment's success rate compared to the expected quality and length of life without the treatment.[5] While the benefits of chemotherapy vary with different types of cancer, one study reported that only 7 percent of all human cancers gain a notable increase in survival time.[6] And, in some cases, traditional cancer treatments produce a negative outcome. The *British Journal of Cancer* published a study involving patients who had undergone surgery for colorectal cancer. One group was treated with chemotherapy, the other received a placebo. For the first five years, survival rates for the two groups were similar, although the chemotherapy group suffered more side effects and a lower quality of life. Beyond the five-year mark, the chemotherapy group showed a sharp increase in deaths, while the group receiving no treatment showed no increase. The placebo group's long-range survival was nearly double that of the chemotherapy group (68 percent vs. 38 percent).[7]

After reading this study, I made a special effort to determine how my own prognosis had been affected by radiation and chemotherapy. I found very little information. (What I did find suggested a greatly increased risk of leukemia and secondary brain tumors.) A paucity of data is understandable for glioblastoma patients, because few survive long enough for a treatment's side effects to become evident. It is much less understandable for breast cancer, prostate cancer, and other cancers having numerous long-term survivors; nevertheless, little information can be found.

Given the high risks and minimal benefits, it is not surprising that practitioners of alternative medicine are critical of mainstream cancer treatments. Few oncologists would dispute the fact that traditional treatments exact a heavy toll with an uncertain benefit; nevertheless, most feel that much alternative medicine is a menace to the patient's well-being. Moreover, alternative treatments are often accompanied by considerable hype, but they lack the scientific evidence to support claims of success. As a result, patients are sometimes seduced away from conventional medicine, which oncologists believe provides the best chance for successful treatment. This seduction is at the heart of conventional medicine's antipathy for alternative medicine. It is not the specific treatments to which oncologists are opposed—these will cease or persist according to their success rate. It is the fact that alternative medicine is embedded in a framework of unscientific analysis, where evidence is anecdotal at best and proponents operate outside the canon of scientific medicine, often in a way that seems financially self-serving.

There has been growing sentiment among physicians that the FDA should actively regulate alternative supplements, using the same standards required for conventional drugs. But various politicians, mainly in the Senate, are sympathetic to alternative medicine and have opposed the extension of FDA control. They also mandated the National Cancer Institute (NCI) to take a more active interest in alternative medicine. As a result, the NCI now has a separate division to fund research on alternative treatments, and has already financed facilities at several major cancer centers, including M.D. Anderson in Houston and Sloan-Kettering in New York. Among the treatments being studied are green tea, mistletoe, ginseng, oleander, melatonin, Flor-Essence (essiac tea), 714X, Chinese herbs, shark cartilage, and dietary regimens for pancreatic cancer.

Some oncologists, including officials at the NCI, strongly opposed the creation of the alternative medicine division. They saw it as a government endorsement of unscientific practices, and they feared it would siphon funds from conventional research. This attitude ignores the fact that many conventional treatments were developed from folk medicine. (Even Taxol, a widely used chemotherapy agent, was derived from the bark of a tree growing in forests along the Pacific coast.) As it has in the past, folklore might provide the groundwork for promising new treatments. There is no reason to debunk these without further investigations, but that is what American medicine typically has done.

Many European and Asian countries have been more receptive to folk remedies; in fact, their physicians frequently prescribe nonpharmaceutical supplements as first-line treatments (for example, St. John's wort for mild cases of depression, or glucosamine for arthritis). Even our northern neighbor, Canada, is more tolerant of alternative medicine. In 1998, the *Canadian Medical Association Journal* reviewed six alternative therapies. While they made no endorsements, the reviewers noted that several of the treatments showed anticancer activity in the laboratory and therefore merited further investigation.

Perspectives on Alternative Treatments

The conflict between conventional and alternative medicine makes it difficult for patients to evaluate nonmainstream treatments. The main problem lies in assessing the credibility of the various sources of information. For example, when members of conventional medicine criticize alternative treatments, alternative practitioners often allege ethical misconduct. Evidence that supposedly discredits their theories is debunked on various grounds, ranging from the incompetence of those conducting clinical trials to the intentional undermining of protocols in order to ensure that treatment effects are not detected. Perhaps the strongest rebuttal has been that studies of individual treatment components are invalid because beneficial interactions are only evident when components are combined.

Patients evaluating alternative treatments need to consider both sides. The following examples illustrate several dimensions of the conflict. The case of alternative medicine is taken primarily from *Alternative Medicine Definitive Guide to Cancer.* Criticisms come primarily from Quackwatch, a Web site presenting conventional medicine's perspective on a number of alternative treatments.[8] Reading these sources side by side, the contrast is stark.

LAETRILE

During the 1970s and early 1980s, laetrile (also known as amygdalin or vitamin B_{17}) achieved great notoriety as an anticancer agent. Today, it is widely regarded as having been discredited. According to Quackwatch, laetrile is not only ineffective, but dangerous: it has reportedly produced lethal cyanide poisoning in some patients.

Evidence that laetrile has no effect on cancer comes from NCI-sponsored clinical trials conducted by Mayo Clinic and three other cancer centers. Patients participating in the trials had advanced cancer for which no proven treatment was known. They were given intravenous laetrile for three weeks, then they were switched to oral laetrile. According to Quackwatch, of 178 patients, none were cured or stabilized, and not one showed a decrease in cancer-related symptoms. Several patients experienced symptoms of cyanide toxicity, with blood levels approaching the lethal range.

Despite this evidence, nine of the twenty-three treatment regimens described in *Alternative Medicine Definitive Guide to Cancer* continue to include laetrile. These practitioners dispute the validity of the Mayo Clinic study, claiming that a relatively inactive form of laetrile was used and that patients were so debilitated that no therapy would have had a long-term effect. They also maintain that 70 percent of the patients had stabilized during the intravenous laetrile; only when intravenous treatment was replaced by oral laetrile did the patients' health decline. They further contend that animal studies supporting the efficacy of laetrile were conducted at Sloan-Kettering Hospital in the 1970s by Dr. Kanematsu Sugiura, but the evidence was suppressed by officials at the cancer center. Dr. Ralph Moss, now a contributor to alternative medicine literature, was discharged because he revealed that authorities had covered up the positive findings. The supposed motive for this cover-up was laetrile's nonpatentability: the positive findings posed a threat to the profits of the pharmaceutical industry, from which Sloan-Kettering derives substantial funds.[9]

All of these allegations have been disputed, and alternative medicine has offered no worthwhile evidence of laetrile's clinical efficacy. This lack of critical scrutiny goes a long way toward justifying the mainstream's dismissal of alternative medicine as snake oil.

HYDRAZINE SULFATE

During the early 1970s, hydrazine sulfate enjoyed considerable interest as an important treatment breakthrough. Developed by Dr. Joseph Gold to treat cachexia (the weight loss and loss of appetite often associated with cancer), it was quickly seen as a potential treatment for the cancer itself.

Hydrazine sulfate interferes with the process by which lactic acid (created by cancer cells) is reconverted back into glucose. According to Dr. Gold's theory, this conversion process requires a great deal of energy, and this energy is captured from the body's normal metabolic process, causing the weight loss. Dr. Gold believed that most cancer patients die not from their cancer, but from the general debilitation associated with cachexia. Thus, by inhibiting the reconversion of lactic acid into glucose, hydrazine sulfate should improve the general health and eventual clinical outcome of cancer patients.

There is no disagreement that cachexia is a factor in a large number of cancer deaths. However, it is debatable whether hydrazine sulfate is an effective treatment for cachexia, and whether it has any meaningful benefit for cancer patients. Several animal studies supported the efficacy of hydrazine sulfate, and clinical studies in Russia reported that 33 percent of cancer patients showed measurable improvements with minimal toxicity.[10,11] But when Sloan-Kettering conducted a clinical trial, it failed to replicate the positive results reported in Russia. Dr. Gold regarded the clinical trial as a deliberate attempt to sabotage the drug: it used much higher dosages than he had recommended, which, he claims, undermined the drug's effectiveness and created considerable toxicity.[12]

Subsequent clinical trials, conducted in the 1980s by Dr. Rowan Chlebowski at UCLA, were more successful.[13] This engendered renewed interest in hydrazine sulfate, resulting in the conduct of three new randomized, placebo-controlled clinical trials. None of them demonstrated clinical efficacy.[14,15,16] Moreover, one of the trials suggested that the drug might have a negative effect, hastening cancer progression and lowering quality of life. Again, Dr. Gold argued that the trials were invalid because the protocols included various substances that interfered with the drug's effect.

According to *Alternative Medicine Definitive Guide to Cancer*, deviations from the recommended protocol were part of a deliberate effort to prevent competition with the pharmaceutical industry. According to Quackwatch, the National Cancer Institute reanalyzed the clinical trial results to assess the role of the supposedly confounding variables, and it found no evidence that these affected the trial's outcome.

ISCADOR

One of the most commonly used supplements in Europe is Iscador, an extract of European mistletoe (a different species than American mistletoe). According to a review by the *Canadian Medical Association Journal*,[17] over 80,000 patients in Switzerland and Germany have been treated with Iscador, often in conjunction with dietary, artistic, and movement therapies derived from the discipline of anthroposophy, first introduced in 1920 by Rudolf Steiner in Austria. According to the anthroposophic medical model, a human being comprises four dimensions of energy that influence and govern all aspects of life: the physical body; the field of life energy surrounding the body; the realm of feelings and emotions; and the ego, the seat of self-awareness and consciousness. Healthy individuals enjoy cooperation between these four dimensions; therefore, cancer, like all diseases, should be considered a disease of the whole person, not a disease of cells.[18]

Anthroposophy views Iscador as promoting these higher-organizing forces, but Quackwatch dismisses Iscador's value, noting that Rudolf Steiner espoused occult beliefs. There is no reason, however, that a remedy so widely used in medical contexts cannot be dissociated from its historical origins. Modern medical practice contains many elements that had questionable beginnings, but this is irrelevant to their utility.

Contrary to the derogatory opinion of Quackwatch, there is substantial evidence from rodent experiments that Iscador is beneficial, including the suppression of over 90 percent of lung metastases from melanoma tumors, and the complete inhibition of carcinogen-induced sarcoma, even with very low dosages.[19,20] The most likely explanation for these effects is that Iscador's main ingredients, iscumen and viscotoxin, are lectins that inhibit protein synthesis and stimulate various cytokines that increase leukocyte count (the white blood cells essential to immune function). Iscador also contains polysaccharides similar to those found in various mushroom extracts (discussed in chapter 13), which may contribute to its effects in various animals.[21] Such effects have also been reported in human clinical trials, including one involving glioma patients:[22] those receiving Iscador plus radiation treatment had a median survival time of twenty months vs. ten months for patients receiving only radiation treatment.[23]

Laboratory research on the therapeutic effects of Iscador has accelerated over the past five years, and a number of papers were presented at the 1999 meeting of the American Association for Cancer Research. Numerous animal studies combined with anecdotal evidence indicate that Iscador is a potential adjunct for cancer treatment and a candidate for further investigation. Moreover, based on its long history of use, there appears to be little risk involved, as the only identified side effect is a mild inflammatory reaction at the site of injection.

Any agent that has an established safety record and strong evidence of boosting the immune system ought to be taken seriously. Because of its historical origins, however, American oncology has paid little attention to the evidence supporting Iscador's clinical utility. This is a prime example of conventional medicine rejecting alternative agents not on the basis of scientific evidence, but because of their association with "unacceptable" approaches to medicine.

UKRAIN

Whereas Iscador is used as an adjunct to the standard cancer treatment, some alternative agents are intended as substitutes for conventional forms of chemotherapy. The most promising of these is Ukrain, which, as the name implies, was developed in the former Soviet Union. There it is regarded not as alternative medicine, but as a form of chemotherapy. It has fewer side effects than conventional chemotherapy and reportedly enhances, rather than harms, the immune system.[24]

Ukrain is of special interest because one of its two ingredients is thiotepa, a highly toxic chemotherapy agent used in bone marrow transplants, where its toxicity makes it effective in killing existing bone marrow cells prior to transplantation. Ukrain's second ingredient, a common plant called celandine, neutralizes the toxicity of thiotepa for normal cells.

Ukrain is believed to increase oxygen consumption in both normal and cancerous cells. After hyperoxidation, the metabolism of normal cells returns to normal while that of cancerous cells ceases altogether, causing them to die. Ukrain is also thought to increase the number of T helper cells, thus boosting the immune system. In an in vitro study of the sixty different cell lines used by the National Cancer Institute to screen potential cancer treatments, moderate dosages of Ukrain inhibited cell growth in fifty-seven lines, and high dosages inhibited growth in all sixty.[25] These results are supported by clinical evidence. Dr. Robert Atkins (inventor of the Atkins Low-Carbohydrate Diet and a contributor to *Alternative Medicine Definitive Guide to Cancer*) reported that forty of the first fifty-two patients he treated with Ukrain received a significant degree of benefit, although he did not elaborate on what this meant.

Two other contributors to *Alternative Medicine Definitive Guide to Cancer* have also included the drug in their treatment protocols, and one reported success in combining Ukrain with Taxol.

Published clinical results for Ukrain consist primarily of case reports, a number of which indicate complete remissions. Case histories include patients with advanced cervical cancer, metastatic breast cancer, esophageal cancer, lung cancer, and metastatic melanoma. Most of these patients reportedly tried and failed the conventional treatments. While case histories provide only weak evidence of treatment efficacy, the fact that complete remissions have occurred in patients with extremely poor prognoses should provoke further investigation. As yet, oncologists in the United States have taken little interest in Ukrain's potential.

One bona fide randomized clinical trial tested Ukrain as a treatment for colorectal carcinoma.[26] The control condition was the standard treatment of 5-fluorouracil and radiation. For patients with metastatic cancer, tumor regression occurred in 40 percent of those treated with Ukrain, while no regression occurred in the control group. For patients with nonmetastatic colorectal cancer, the twenty-month survival rate was 79 percent for the Ukrain group and only 33 percent for those given the conventional treatment. A second randomized clinical trial investigated the effects of Ukrain in the treatment of pancreatic cancer.[27] Patients received 5.4 g/day vitamin C plus either saline injections or Ukrain. The one-year survival rate was 81 percent in the Ukrain group compared with 14 percent in the control group. The two-year survival rate was 43 percent in the Ukrain group vs. 5 percent in the control group. Median survival time was seventeen months for patients who received Ukrain and seven months for those who did not. The typical median survival for pancreatic cancer patients is six to eight months.

It seems there is no question that Ukrain should be considered a treatment option. Further study will more clearly define its degree of effectiveness for different kinds of cancer.

OTHER TREATMENTS

These examples offer only a flavor of the treatments endorsed by alternative medicine. A more comprehensive introduction would include essiac tea, Cantron, 714x, Coley's toxin, and a variety of others. For more information about these and other treatments, consult *Alternative Medicine Definitive Guide to Cancer.* For the perspective of conventional medicine, go to quackwatch.com. There is almost no overlap between the two.

From my own perspective, many treatments are not as far-fetched as conventional medicine would have us believe, though supporting evidence is far from convincing. For example, Quackwatch dismisses the idea that a generalized immunological reaction to a toxin or virus may provide an effective cancer treatment; however, a number of studies contradict this. Brain tumor patients who contract postsurgical infections appear to have an improved prognosis, suggesting that the immune system's response to the infectious agent sensitizes the immune system to the cancer cells. At least some evidence from clinical trials supports this idea.

In the early 1990s, for example, phase-II clinical trials tested the toxin ImuVert (the biological extract of *Serratia marcescens*) against recurrent gliomas.[28] Although only a small percentage of patients exhibited a measurable response, three of nineteen patients enjoyed long-term survival. Another example comes from the study of Newcastle disease, which is fatal to chickens but apparently has no adverse effect on normal human cells. For cancer cells, on the other hand, there is evidence that the Newcastle disease vaccine has a potent cytotoxic effect.[29] In a small but randomized clinical trial, thirty-three patients with various types of advanced cancer received either the vaccine or a placebo. No regressions were seen in the placebo group, but tumor regression occurred for eight patients who received the vaccine, seven of whom were still alive after a two-year follow-up. The only side effect was a slight fever in a minority of patients. More impressive results have been reported using the Newcastle virus to treat melanoma: patients with stage-III melanoma who received the vaccine postsurgically had a ten-year survival rate over 60 percent.[30]

There is even stronger evidence supporting the clinical efficacy of various herbal treatments. Consider an herbal concoction known as SPES, which was developed by a court physician for a Chinese emperor to treat urinary and prostate problems. I first learned of SPES from an uncle who had prostate cancer. When he added SPES to his assortment of herbal and vitamin supplements, his elevated PSA count (prostate specific antigen count, which indicates the degree of prostate cancer activity) dropped to near zero. After some investigation, I learned that SPES had become so popular it was being studied by conventional medicine. In one trial, 82 percent of patients receiving SPES—including a significant number who had become insensitive to the standard androgen suppression treatment—experienced reduced PSA levels within two months, and 88 percent had reduced PSA counts after twelve months, which indicates that the treatment did not lose its effectiveness over time.[31] Side effects were comparable to those caused by estrogen treatment, including a higher risk of blood clots and a loss of libido. Similar results have been reported in a number of cancer journals.

Because there are few alternatives for patients who no longer respond to androgen-suppressive therapies, SPES likely will become a standard treatment for prostate cancer. My hope is that other promising alternative treatments will also receive serious attention from conventional medicine.

Conventional vs. Alternative Medicine

Any new treatment advanced by alternative medicine must overcome a catch-22: On the one hand, no treatment will be adopted unless it has met the standards set by conventional medicine. On the other hand, agents not backed by the medical and pharmaceutical communities do not generate the resources necessary for a serious study to be conducted. In other words, you have to play by the rules, but they won't let you play without a ticket. This fuels much of the resentment that alternative medicine has shown toward conventional medical practice. Based on their clinical experience, alternative practitioners are convinced they are using effective treatments, and they appear willing to conduct small clinical trials to support their contentions. Nevertheless, they can't seem to interest the larger medical community. This does not mean that advocates of conventional medicine are deviously undermining alternative medicine. It merely reflects the entrenchment of conventional standards, even when they are not well thought out. As noted in chapter 8, the first principle of the Hippocratic oath is to maintain the requirements for membership in the medical guild. Modern conventional medicine is simply following a well-trodden path.

The Burzynski Case

An example of the contingencies attached to membership in the medical guild is the case of Stanislaw Burzynski, father of the antineoplaston treatment for cancer. After four separate attempts by the U.S. government to prosecute him for criminal offenses, followed by a backlash of support from his patients that eventually resulted in testimony before Congress, Burzynski is regarded as a hero by much of the cancer community. His case has now attained epic proportions.

Prize-winning journalist Thomas D. Elias presents an excellent account of Burzynski's story in *The Burzynski Breakthrough and the Government's Campaign to Squelch It*.[32] Stanislaw Burzynski is a medical researcher who received both an MD and PhD from the leading medical university in Poland. In his doctoral dissertation, published in 1968, Burzynski described the differences between the amino acids of kidney disease patients and those of healthy patients. He hypothesized that these differences might be important in understanding cancer. Burzynski had observed that patients with kidney disease seldom develop cancer, and that cancer patients often lack several key amino acids. Because a function of the kidneys is to filter amino acids from the blood, he inferred that the kidneys of cancer patients remove amino acids that are important for cancer prevention.

At first, Burzynski's research was well received by Polish authorities, and he was actively recruited to join the Communist Party. He declined because his own family had been persecuted by the Communist government and his brother was actively involved in the resistance movement. Soon thereafter his brother was arrested (and presumably murdered) and Burzynski received a draft notice. He immediately left Poland for the United States, bringing with him a distrust for Big Brother government and a proclivity to resist its intrusion into his scientific work.

Upon arriving in the United States, Burzynski obtained a first-rate academic position at Baylor University in Houston, Texas, working under Dr. George Unger in anesthesiology. He spent half his time on projects directed by Unger and half pursuing independent research on amino acids. During this time, Burzynski developed a theory that would guide his future efforts: cancer cells grow out of control because they lack amino acids necessary for normal cell division; thus, providing these amino acids will restore normal cell division and differentiation.

Burzynski received a promotion and a pay raise, as well as a grant from the National Cancer Institute to pursue his research. He began by distilling what he believed to be the critical amino acids from his own urine, then testing these in cultures of different cancer cells. He saw considerable variation in the anticancer potency of the different amino acids, so he concentrated his efforts on those that were most effective. These he named antineoplastons, derived from *neoplasm,* the Greek term for cancerous tumors.

BATTLING THE FDA

Burzynski's transformation from rising star to medical pariah occurred when he attempted to use his antineoplaston treatment with human patients at Baylor University. To do so, he required an IND (a permit for an investigational new drug) approved by both Baylor and the FDA. He had met the first criterion, demonstrating that antineoplaston treatment was effective in cell cultures of human cancers. But he failed to meet the second criterion: demonstrating that the treatment was effective in animal models (usually implanted with tumors derived from human cell lines). In fact, the antineoplastons had shown little effect in animal experiments. According to Burzynski, this is because peptides manufactured by animals to control cancer cells are species-specific. Whether or not this is true,[33] he was unable to obtain an IND from either Baylor or the FDA.

Not to be deterred, Burzynski convinced a local community hospital, unaffiliated with the major medical schools, to let him test his treatment on terminally ill patients. This decision to operate outside the rules of the medical establishment was the first step to professional ostracism and eventual prosecution.

Soon, Burzynski faced a critical decision that would determine the path of his career. His sponsor, George Unger, left his position in the anesthesiology department, forcing Burzynski to find his own way. Baylor invited Burzynski to become a full-time member of the Baylor Cancer Research Center, with the condition that he give up his private medical practice. This offer would have given Burzynski professional prestige and security, but his laboratory space and in-house grant support would have decreased, because the cancer center did not have the same level of funding as the anesthesiology department.

Burzynski declined. Perhaps, after his experiences in Poland, he did not want to submit to the authority of an institution. As long as he had a private medical practice, he could use whatever medications he thought would be effective, subject only to the consent of his patients. But the future would not be so simple.

Burzynski terminated his affiliation with Baylor University in 1977. For the next few years, he manufactured his most promising antineoplastons and used them in his private medical practice. Several of his success stories received considerable publicity, and it was not long before his "unproven treatment" had gained the attention of medical authorities.

In 1983, the FDA filed a lawsuit with the stated intention of shutting down his one-man operation. Even before the suit could be heard, the FDA asked for a temporary injunction to stop Burzynski's activities. In fact, the agency had no jurisdiction except as granted by the Interstate Commerce Act: as long as Burzynski did not ship his medications across state lines, the federal government was powerless to stop him. Predictably, the judge ordered Burzynski to stop shipping and selling antineoplastons across state lines until they were approved by the FDA, and to bring his manufacturing process in compliance with good manufacturing practice. The judge also made it clear that nothing about his ruling should be construed as an order to prevent Burzynski from using his medication in Texas.

For the next decade, the FDA continued its attempts to prosecute Burzynski. On two occasions it convinced government authorities to convene a grand jury, but charges were never filed. The FDA's persistence, however, eventually paid off, resulting in two separate criminal trials. The first ended in a hung jury, the second in acquittal. Throughout, Burzynski was charged with profiteering and violating the court's injunction against selling his antineoplastons across state lines. At no time was the efficacy of Burzynski's treatment an issue. Instead, because the treatment had not been certified by the FDA, it was ipso facto illegal, regardless of its efficacy.

There is no doubt that Burzynski treated patients from other states, but they were first required to come to Houston for an evaluation and instructions about administering the treatment. When prolonged stays in Houston were impossible, patients received their medications by mail, but not directly from Burzynski. Instead, the patients' friends or relatives acquired the drugs from Burzynski, so he thought he was relieved of responsibility for what was otherwise considered a criminal action.

The FDA's profiteering charge was apparently based on the high cost of Burzynski's treatment. While various amounts have been quoted, a number of sources estimate that it was $10,000 per month. Of course, conventional cancer treatments often are just as expensive, and some, such as bone marrow transplants, are many times more expensive. It is also important to recognize the high cost of Burzynski's business. He received no support from any kind of governmental agency, he faced increasing difficulty in getting insurance companies to cover his treatment, and he accommodated more and more patients who sought his assistance. All of this required large and expensive operations. The profiteering charge was especially ironic given the FDA's open sanction of profiteering by American pharmaceutical companies. Drugs produced by American companies are notably cheaper in every other country in the world, with the difference being as much as ten to one. The drug companies and the FDA argue that this markup provides necessary funds for basic research and drug development. Why should Burzynski's operations be viewed any differently?

The FDA's relentless attempts to prosecute Burzynski cost the government millions of dollars. Throughout the ordeal, Burzynski received great support from his patients, including demonstrations outside the courtroom and letter-writing campaigns to government officials. This eventually led to congressional hearings at which FDA officials, Burzynski, and several of his patients testified. Congress was not pleased with the FDA's conduct. Indeed, Congressman Richard Burr, a member of the hearing committee, made an extraordinary condemnation: "The FDA's abuse of power transcends regulatory misconduct. It constitutes nothing less than one of the worst abuses of the criminal justice system I have ever witnessed."

The FDA bowed to political pressure and granted Burzynski an IND. Burzynski is currently conducting clinical trials, the results of which will be reported to the FDA. Only time will tell whether the treatment will be successful.

CONFLICTING EVIDENCE FOR ANTINEOPLASTON TREATMENT

There is an extraordinary contrast between Elias' account of Burzynski's treatment and the perspective offered by Quackwatch, which perhaps represents the general sentiment of conventional medicine. In its 1996 summary of questionable cancer therapies, Quackwatch disputed Burzynski's claim to have helped many cancer patients. It referred readers to a 1992 paper published by Saul Green in *Journal of the American Medical Association*, which concluded that none of Burzynski's drugs have been shown to normalize tumor cells. Quackwatch also noted that legal actions against Burzynski were presumptive evidence of misconduct. It went on to report that six patients died soon after they sought his treatment, though it presented no details about their diagnoses.

Much of this "evidence" offers no foundation for evaluating Burzynski's treatment. The paper by Saul Green is more interesting, as it provides a basis for the quasi-official opinion about Burzynski. Thomas Elias considers the Green article in detail, concluding that it was extremely biased and paid little attention to the evidence pertinent to Burzynski's treatment. Elias' opinion is supported by an in-house review conducted by Dr. Lichuan Chen for the Office of Alternative Medicine at the National Institutes of Health. Chen described many of Green's statements as "misrepresentations and misinterpretations," concluding that Burzynski's work is credible and deserves further study.

Although it is unclear just how effective Burzynski's treatment will be, it clearly warrants meaningful investigation. In preparation for the first criminal trial, Burzynski's lawyers asked Dr. Robert Burdick, a respected oncologist at the University of Washington Medical School, to evaluate the case histories of seventeen patients treated by Burzynski. Burdick's report was not entered into evidence, because the judge ruled that the efficacy of antineoplastons was not pertinent to the case. This ruling was unfortunate, as Burdick's assessment would have cast a different light on Burzynski's credibility. It noted that Burzynski's treatments had been remarkably successful: of the seventeen cases reviewed, there were seven complete remissions, nine partial remissions of 50 percent or more, and one patient with stable disease.

Support also comes from the National Cancer Institute (NCI). In keeping with a new policy, the NCI sent a review panel to visit Burzynski's clinic and evaluate his best outcomes. Burzynski presented the case histories of twenty brain tumor patients, but the review panel examined only seven, citing time constraints. Despite the limited number of cases, the panel determined that antitumor activity was clearly documented.

A third piece of support comes from a review by independent radiologists at the Southwest Neuro-Imaging Center in Phoenix. Of twenty-eight brain tumor patients treated by Burzynski, thirteen had their tumors shrink by more than 50 percent, and three more showed significant improvement that was less than 50 percent.

Clinical trials have only added to the controversy. The first trial, sponsored by the National Cancer Institute and involving brain tumors, was reported in *Mayo Clinic Proceedings*.[34] The results for only nine patients were published, which precludes any definite conclusion about treatment efficacy. The nine patients showed no evidence of tumor regression, and several suffered toxic side effects from the treatment. These results appear quite damaging to Burzynski's claims, but there were several irregularities in the conduct of the trial, suggesting that it may not have been a fair test of antineoplastons.

The trial was terminated early, after Burzynski objected to a change in the eligibility criteria for patients. The change was made because not enough patients could be recruited under the original criteria. One wonders how problems in patient recruitment could occur, given that hundreds of patients were willing to travel thousands of miles and pay many thousands of dollars to receive Burzynski's treatment. Why were

SURVIVING "TERMINAL" CANCER

major cancer centers—the National Institutes of Health, Mayo Clinic, and Sloan-Kettering—unable to generate interest when the treatment was free?

An examination of the patients' histories suggests that potential trial participants were advised to seek other treatments unless their case was hopeless. Furthermore, most participants had one or two treatments between initial tumor recurrence and antineoplaston treatment, and the time before the next recurrence was quite brief, indicating highly aggressive tumors. Even then, the median survival time after antineoplaston treatment was approximately seven months, hardly impressive but still superior to the four-to-six months typical of other treatments. Moreover, three of the nine patients lived for one year or longer. Thus, the claim that the treatment showed no effect in clinical trials was misleading.

The absence of tumor regression in the NCI studies runs counter to Burzynski's retrospective report, published in *Clinical Drug Investigation*.[35] Of thirty-six patients with recurrent primary brain tumors, sixteen had a complete or partial response. Eleven were still alive when the report was published, having an average survival of 5.5 years from the start of antineoplaston therapy. Another four patients with stable disease were also still alive, with an average survival of 3.5 years. These results are difficult to interpret because they are not broken down by diagnostic category. Only fourteen patients had glioblastomas, and their outcomes were unclear. Nevertheless, the results suggest that antineoplastons may have a meaningful degree of effectiveness.

Burzynski also released an annual report, detailing the patients he treated in 1997, to *The Cancer Letter*, the organization that publishes Quackwatch. *The Cancer Letter* commissioned three independent reviewers to evaluate Burzynski's results. For the brain tumor patients, the reviewer was Dr. Henry Friedman of Duke University, a neuro-oncologist for whom I have great respect.

Friedman's evaluation was harsh, to say the least. Part of his criticism related to Burzynski's procedures: he had left out critical details, such as how adherence to the protocols was verified and at what points patient outcome was assessed. More importantly, Friedman was unconvinced that Burzynski's interpretation of the MRIs was correct. As Friedman noted, there are numerous factors involved in distinguishing changes in a tumor from other variables that affect an MRI, including changes in steroid level and residual scar tissue from surgery and radiation, which may resolve on their own regardless of the treatment. It is unfair, however, to say that Burzynski's assessment depended solely on his interpretation of the MRIs. In fact, Burzynski had submitted his records, including successive MRIs, to independent reviewers on three occasions. In every case, the reviewers concurred with Burzynski, and some of their evaluations were even more positive.

Friedman also noted his grave concern about the potential toxicity of antineoplastons, especially for brain tumor patients. The drugs cause high sodium levels that can aggravate edema. Given that brain tumor patients often die from intracranial pressure, this represents a serious threat. Burzynski has attempted to answer this concern on several occasions, noting that high sodium levels and increased edema quickly resolve themselves if the patient drinks enough water to remain properly hydrated.

It is important to note that Friedman did not claim Burzynski's treatment was ineffective, only that its effects were so sloppily reported that they were not interpretable. He also encouraged a longer follow-up period to allow a better evaluation of survival times.

What is a brain tumor patient to make of the incredible controversy surrounding Burzynski's treatment? Should antineoplastons be considered an option? In my opinion, the treatment has at least some efficacy, and MRI evaluations by outside reviewers support this conclusion. At the same time, patients need more information: effectiveness has not been specified for different types of brain tumors. Burzynski lumped the diagnostic categories together, then made a case for antineoplaston therapy by describing the dismal prognosis and lack of effective treatment for brain tumors in general. While such an assessment is true for glioblastomas, conventional treatments have considerable benefits for lower-grade tumors. For example, patients with grade-III astrocytomas have a median survival time of almost four years when treated with conventional chemotherapy (usually PCV). Oligodendrogliomas also respond well to chemotherapy. Perhaps the most dramatic results were seen in a phase-II trial where patients with anaplastic astrocytomas were given Poly-ICLC; all but one were alive after five years.[36]

Clearly, for many brain tumors, there are treatment options other than Burzynski's. But this is not the case for glioblastomas. If Burzynski's success rate with glioblastomas is anywhere near the numbers he has quoted for brain tumors in general, his antineoplastons will assume center stage. But without a more detailed report of his results, the case will not be made.

Separating Fact from Fiction

The Burzynski case illustrates the conflict between conventional and alternative medicine. The latter category is so amorphous that its treatments have little in common—other than the fact that conventional medicine views them as unproven and unacceptable. But as we have seen, many alternative treatments have promise. It is a mistake to dismiss them simply because they do not conform to the rules practiced by conventional medicine. In doing so, mainstream medicine shows more concern about maintaining hegemony over medical practice than improving patient outcome. If Burzynski's treatment turns out to be effective for glioblastomas, its oppression by the conventional medical establishment, and especially the FDA, will be remembered as one of the most self-serving episodes in medical history. Due to his incomplete reporting, Burzynski is certainly responsible for some of the negative response his work has received. But the issue is not who will win the contest between Burzynski and his critics. It is how to maximize the benefits for cancer patients. Whether conventional medicine can be trusted to serve this higher purpose is questionable.

While conventional and alternative practitioners continue their feud, cancer patients must sift through conflicting information. They will find that some alternative treatments, like laetrile, have no supporting evidence, while the benefits of others, like Iscador and Ukrain, are well documented. The majority of treatments, however, are less clear-cut. Many begin with a plausible rationale for why they work, along with laboratory research that provides at least some support for their efficacy. Often, these treatments are widely used in other countries, though usage may be based on case histories rather than controlled clinical trials. Such usage may inspire clinical trials in the United States, where the treatments frequently fail to show efficacy. Proponents of alternative medicine then reject the clinical trials, alleging an active conspiracy between the pharmaceutical industry and conventional medicine.

As discussed in previous chapters, conventional medicine's rigid distinction between proven and unproven treatments is unjustifiable. There are many ways to produce a negative result in a clinical trial, even when the treatment is efficacious. This does not mean there is a villain behind every tree deliberately attempting to undermine the clinical trials. In the case of hydrazine sulfate, the three trials conducted subsequent to the positive results of Dr. Chlebowski were totally persuasive. None of them offered even a hint of benefit from hydrazine sulfate, as the small numerical difference between the treatment and control groups was in favor of the control.

The fact that some alternative treatments can be persuasively rejected provides no justification for the broad-stroke denigration of alternative medicine. First, failure in phase-III clinical trials does not mean a treatment is ineffective. Second, conventional cancer treatments have not been successful enough to preclude other promising treatments simply because they lie outside the mainstream. When even a few glioblastoma patients are reportedly cured by a new treatment, that treatment should be taken seriously. Almost any alternative with even a modicum of evidence seems preferable to conventional treatments that have a known record of failure.

ENDNOTES

1. Diamond, W. J., Cowden, W. L., and Goldberg, B. *Alternative Medicine Definitive Guide to Cancer.* Tiburon, Calif.: Future Medicine Publishing, Inc.; 1997.

2. It is important to appreciate that case histories are the natural method for reporting data when idiosyncratic treatment plans are developed for individual patients. To their credit, practitioners of alternative medicine have ignored standard procedures for proving treatment efficacy because they believe that most of the evidence emerges at the individual patient level. While most oncologists agree that age, level of functioning, and other variables will affect a patient's outcome, conventional medicine ignores the possibility that individual differences may also determine the effect of the treatment. This is a failing of traditional medicine. In contrast, alternative medicine believes that patient-treatment interactions may be as important, if not more important, in determining treatment outcome than the type of treatment itself.

3. This is the major complaint against alternative medicine. Unless practitioners keep and report good records for all their patients, critics have every right to challenge any claims that are made. If alternative medicine expects to be taken seriously, a treatment scorecard is essential. For deadly cancers such as glioblastoma, pancreatic cancer, and most types of advanced metastatic cancer, a documented success rate may serve as reasonable evidence of a treatment's efficacy, even if no two patients receive the same treatment protocol.

4. As adjuncts to conventional treatment, these therapies appear relatively benign, and many people view them as complementary medicine rather than alternative medicine. Nevertheless, some of these treatments have been controversial. For example, many experts believe that antioxidants should be avoided when the patient is undergoing radiation and chemotherapy. We will consider this issue in the next chapter, along with recommendations about which supplements are most likely to be useful.

5. Different stages of cancer have very different prognoses. When cancer is in an early stage, it often can be completely resected and the survival rate is high as a result. With advanced, metastatic cancer, surgery is no longer an option and typically only chemotherapy is used. The problem with relating cancer survival rates to various treatments is that different stages of cancer are often reported as an aggregate. For patients deciding whether or not to undergo chemotherapy, such aggregate statistics are not helpful. The essential information is the survival rate or increase in longevity when chemotherapy is the only option. For most cancers, few patients with late-stage disease are helped by chemotherapy.

6. Diamond, W. J., Cowden, W. L., and Goldberg, B. *Alternative Medicine Definitive Guide to Cancer.* Tiburon, Calif.: Future Medicine Publishing, Inc.; 1997:845.

7. Chlebowski, R. T., et al. Late mortality and levamisole adjuvant therapy of resected colon carcinoma. *British Journal of Cancer.* 1994;69:1094-1097.

8. Quackwatch (www.quackwatch.com) is maintained primarily by Dr. Stephen Barrett, a frequent contributor to medical books on the topic of alternative medicine.

9. Diamond, W. J., Cowden, W. L., and Goldberg, B. *Alternative Medicine Definitive Guide to Cancer.* Tiburon, Calif.: Future Medicine Publishing Inc.; 1997:673-674.

10. Diamond, W. J., Cowden, W. L., and Goldberg, B. *Alternative Medicine Definitive Guide to Cancer.* Tiburon, Calif.: Future Medicine Publishing, Inc.; 1997:667-673.

11. Filov, V. A., et al. Experience of the treatment with Sehydrin (hydrazine sulfate, HS) in advanced cancer patients. *Investigational New Drugs.* 1995;13(1):89-97.

12. Diamond, W. J., Cowden, W. L., and Goldberg, B. *Alternative Medicine Definitive Guide to Cancer.* Tiburon, Calif.: Future Medicine Publishing, Inc.; 1997:671-672.

13. Chlebowski, R. T., et al. Hydrazine sulfate influence on nutritional status and survival in non-small cell lung cancer. *Journal of Clinical Oncology.* 1990;8(1):9-15.

14. Loprinzi, C. L., et al. Randomized placebo-controlled evaluation of hydrazine sulfate in patients with advanced colorectal cancer. *Journal of Clinical Oncology.* 1994;12(6):1121-1125.

15. Kosty, M. P., et al. Cisplatin, vinblastine, and hydrazine sulfate in advanced, non-small cell lung cancer: a randomized placebo-controlled, double-blind phase-III study of the Cancer and Leukemia Group B. *Journal of Clinical Oncology.* 1994;12(6):1113-1120.

16. Loprinzi, C. L., et al. Placebo-controlled trial of hydrazine sulfate in patients with newly diagnosed non-small cell lung cancer. *Journal of Clinical Oncology.* 1994;12(6):1126-1129.

17. Kaegi, E. Unconventional therapies for cancer: 3 Iscador. Task Force on Alternative Therapies of the Canadian Breast Cancer Research Initiative. *Canadian Medical Association Journal.* 1998;158(9):1157-1159.

18. Stripped of its metaphysical overtones, this is the perspective of holistic medicine in general. It takes seriously the concept of mind-body interactions and believes that nonphysical forces help control bodily functions. This perspective is antithetical to the purely naturalistic view that all bodily processes can be understood in terms of the laws of biology. To modern medicine, there is no ghost in the machine.

Various psychological manipulations can affect our health. For example, stress can induce hypertension or suppress the immune system, and Pavlovian and operant conditioning can cause the release of hormones that affect bodily processes. Though such effects are created by psychological variables, this does not mean that nonphysical forces are involved. These effects are ultimately due to changes in the nervous system, which regulates physiological processes. There is no "mind" that stands outside the nervous system telling it what to do.

19. Kuttan, G., et al. Anticarcinogenic and antimetastatic activity of Iscador. *Anti-cancer Drugs.* 1997 April;8(suppl 1):15S-16S.

20. Antony, S., et al. Effect of *Viscum album* in the inhibition of lung metastasis in mice induced by B16F10 melanoma cells. *Journal of Experimental and Clinical Cancer Research.* 1997;16(2):159-162.

21. Kuttan, G., and Kuttan R. Reduction of leukopenia in mice by *Viscum album* administration during radiation and chemotherapy. *Tumori.* 1993;79(1):74-76.

22. Lenartz, D., et al. Immunoprotective activity of the galactoside-specific lectin from mistletoe after tumor destructive therapy in glioma patients. *Anticancer Research.* 1996;6B:3799-3802.

23. Lenartz, D., et al. Survival of glioma patients after complementary treatment with galactoside-specific lectin from mistletoe. *Anticancer Research.* 2000;20(3B):2073-2076.

24. Jagiello-Woftowicz, E., et al. Ukrain (NSC-631570) in experimental and clinical studies: a review. *Drugs under Experimental Clinical Research.* 1998;24(5-6):213-219.

25. Liepins, A. Ukrain as an experimental cytotoxic agent. *Journal of Chemotherapy.* 1992;5(suppl):797-799.

26. Susak, Y. M., et al. Comparison of chemotherapy and x-ray therapy with Ukrain monotherapy for colorectal cancer. *Drugs under Experimental and Clinical Research.* 1996;22(3-5):115-122.

27. Zemskov, V. S., et al. Ukrain (NSC-631570) in the treatment of pancreas cancer. *Drugs under Experimental Clinical Research.* 2000;26(5-6):179-190.

28. Jaeckle, K. A., et al. Phase-II trial of *Serratia marcescens* extract in recurrent malignant astrocytoma. *Journal of Clinical Oncology.* 1990;8(9):1408-1418.

29. Csatary, L., et al. Attenuated veterinary virus vaccine for the treatment of cancer. *Cancer Detection and Prevention.* 1993;17(6):619-627.

30. Batliwalla, F. M., et al. A 15-year follow-up of AJCC stage-III malignant melanoma patients treated postsurgically with Newcastle disease virus (NDV) oncolysate and determination of alternations in the CD8 T-cell repertoire. *Molecular Medicine.* 1998;4(12):783-794.

31. de la Taille, A., et al. Herbal therapy PC-SPES: in vitro effects and evaluation of its efficacy in 69 patients with prostate cancer. *Journal of Urology.* 2000;164(4):1229-1234.

32. Elias, Thomas D. *The Burzynski Breakthrough and the Government's Campaign to Squelch It.* Santa Monica, Calif.: General Publishing Group; 1997.

33. A study in Taiwan reported major regressions of implanted hepatoma tumors in mice due to distilled human urine. (Lai, G. M., et al. Human urine extracts [CDA-2] as a novel anticancer agent in the aspects of induction of differentiation and apoptosis, antitumorigenesis, chemoprevention, and reversal of drug resistance. *Proceedings of the American Association of Cancer Research.* 1999;abstract 0727.

34. Buckner, J. C., et al. Phase-II study of antineoplastons A10 (NSC648539) and As2-1 (NSC620261) in patients with recurrent glioma. *Mayo Clinic Proceedings.* 1999;74(2):137-145.

35. Burzynski, S. R., et al. A retrospective study of antineoplastons A10 and As2-1 in primary brain tumors. *Clinical Drug Investigation.* 1999;18(1):1-10.

36. See chapter 2, note 6.

The Value of Supplements

CHAPTER THIRTEEN

Found in health-food stores, grocery stores, and drugstores, supplements have grown into a major industry. Several pharmaceutical companies have separate divisions devoted to "nutriceuticals," which include the usual assortment of vitamins and minerals as well as the full gamut of herbal remedies. More than half of cancer patients use supplements, occasionally to the exclusion of conventional treatment. More typically, supplements are used to enhance conventional treatments and ease side effects.

Before discussing popular supplements, there are two general issues to be considered. First is the distinction between cancer prevention and cancer treatment. Many alternative practitioners assume that if an agent is shown to reduce the risk of cancer, it should also be effective in treating cancer. In fact, there is no necessary relationship between the two effects.

For example, antioxidants are known to reduce cancer risk, but they may also interfere with cancer treatments. Various alternative protocols, however, combine antioxidants (such as coenzyme Q_{10} and vitamin E) with gamma-linolenic acid (GLA), which is believed to produce high levels of free radicals. (Recall that GLA is nontoxic to normal cells but highly toxic to cancer cells.) Laboratory experiments have shown that antioxidants may neutralize these free radicals, effectively reducing the anticancer benefits of GLA.

The second issue to consider is that the use of supplements is supported by evidence of variable quality. The weakest and most common form of evidence is epidemiological. For example, Asians have a lower incidence of cancer than Europeans. The fact that Asians consume more soy products has been taken as evidence that soy is an effective anticancer agent and therefore should be incorporated into everyone's diet. There is much to be said in favor of this recommendation. But it is important to recognize that epidemiological evidence is inherently weak. There are always other factors at work, making causal inference impossible. For example, Asians and Europeans also differ in their consumption of red meat, green tea, and other substances. At best, epidemiological evidence can encourage further exploration in controlled settings.

A notch above epidemiological evidence are studies in which subjects record their dietary practices. The differences are then correlated with cancer incidence. Of these, the famous Framingham study is the best known, having tested the effects of coffee, alcohol, and other substances on human health. Results quickly find their way into the media but are usually presented in overly simplistic terms. Often, the public does not see that evidence is based on correlations that may not reflect causal relationships. As a result, newspapers, magazines, and television are filled with new findings that are soon contradicted by other findings, leaving the public in despair of ever learning which dietary practices are beneficial or harmful.

Yet another level of evidence comes from experiments using cultured cancer cells in the laboratory. If an agent retards the growth of these cancer cells, it becomes a serious candidate for clinical trials. But there are many pitfalls along the way. The most common relate to dosage: Is it possible to reach a high enough dosage in patients to replicate the cytotoxicity seen in laboratory studies? This is especially a concern for agents taken orally, as these may be drastically changed by the digestive system. Shark cartilage, for example, has been widely used in alternative medicine because it possesses antiangiogenic properties. At present, antiangiogenesis is the most promising approach to cancer treatment and may even provide a cure. But this does not mean that shark cartilage is an effective treatment for cancer. Critics note that the complex proteins that inhibit angiogenesis are digested when taken orally, so effectiveness in the laboratory is unlikely to translate to effectiveness in the clinic.

A stronger form of laboratory evidence comes from experiments using animals implanted with human cancer cells. Assuming that dosage levels required to produce effects in mice are comparable to those needed for humans, such evidence may support a treatment's efficacy. But even here there are pitfalls. First, drugs are cleared from the body by the liver and kidneys, but different animals will clear a drug at different rates. Also, rodents used in most cancer experiments have a suppressed immune system, allowing an implanted tumor to grow without being rejected by the animal's body. The implications of using immune-suppressed subjects are uncertain.

Because treatments that work in animal experiments may or may not work with humans, we have to try them with humans to find out. But animal experiments at least provide a starting point for sorting out potential treatments. If a substance is highly effective—and nontoxic—in animals, it is not unreasonable to try it as a cancer treatment in humans, even when data from clinical trials are unavailable. If the cost, in terms of potential harm, is minimal, then it is worthwhile to try an agent that might produce a benefit.

Although a majority of supplements are supported only by epidemiological or laboratory evidence, it is a mistake to discount their value. A number of these have shown positive results in bona fide clinical trials, and it is just a matter of time before more evidence becomes available, given that the National Institutes of Health now supports this research.

The Life Extension Foundation

To date, the research on nutritional supplements has been slow because conventional medicine is reluctant to take it seriously. Cancer patients cannot wait for clear-cut evidence, and they must make decisions using the information available.

Several academic journals, including *Nutrition and Cancer, Cancer Letters,* and *Journal of Nutrition,* provide information about the use of dietary supplements in both animal experiments and clinical trials. Unfortunately, most cancer patients are unable to spend time at a medical school library researching this information, and their physicians, if aware of the new findings, are unlikely to share them. As a result, patients get most of their information from suppliers of supplements or from other patients. While much of this is of poor quality (and often bogus), there are some suppliers that appear to be trustworthy. From my own experience, the most valuable information has come from The Life Extension Foundation, which publishes a monthly magazine filled with empirical studies on various supplements. The Life Extension Foundation is a nonprofit organization with an impressive array of physicians on its advisory board. Membership is well worth its modest cost. In addition to the monthly magazine, members receive a substantial discount on supplements that appear to be the highest quality in the industry.[1]

The Life Extension Foundation provides another valuable function: legally challenging the FDA's attempts to overreach its authority. Of special importance has been its battle to prevent the FDA from banning the import of drugs that are essentially the same as those produced by American pharmaceutical companies. A typical case involved Hydergine, which protects and enhances neurological function. Whereas European suppliers offer the drug for less than $20, an equivalent amount costs about $175 in the United States. The FDA's ban on the drug was predicated on the charge that the European version was impure and not up to American quality standards. The Life Extension Foundation made its own analysis and found that the European version actually exceeded American pharmaceutical standards.[2]

The foundation offers a balanced discussion about the value of various supplements, including the theoretical mechanisms by which they work and detailed references to help readers decide if the information is valid. It is often critical of supplements advocated by other members of the alternative medicine community, a notable example being its rejection of shark cartilage based on a survey of members who have used it. The organization seldom overstates its claims. Instead, it allows patients to evaluate supplements after seeing the entire spectrum of evidence, not just clinical trials from conventional medicine.

Luckily for cancer patients, most of these agents are classified not as drugs, but as nutritional supplements. This is an artificial distinction, but one that is important because it limits the FDA's jurisdiction to quality control. Rather than regulating evidence of efficacy, the FDA's role is restricted to preventing suppliers from making unproven claims. This means that many helpful nutritional supplements are available to any cancer patient who is willing to track them down.

The following pages discuss supplements that have a reasonable likelihood of benefiting cancer patients. Many of these are supported by human clinical trials, others have only been studied with animals. Some have evidence of efficacy as preventative agents rather than treatments, a boundary that is often blurred for people who are at high risk of cancer (for example, people with intestinal polyps or a family history of breast cancer).

Vitamin Supplements and Antioxidants

A number of alternative practitioners use mega-dosages of vitamins in their cancer protocols. Most common is vitamin C, where intravenous dosages up to 50 g/day are recommended. The rationale for using vitamin C dates back to the mid-1970s, when two-time Nobel laureate Linus Pauling and Scottish physician Ewan Cameron published a study of one hundred terminal cancer patients treated with 10,000 mg/day of vitamin C. According to their results, these patients lived three to four times longer than similar patients who did not receive vitamin C.[3] Patients in the two groups were not randomly assigned, and critics maintained that the study's results were biased because those who received the vitamin C were Dr. Cameron's patients while those who did not were treated by other physicians. Moreover, they maintained that Cameron labeled his patients "terminal" at an earlier stage in disease than the other physicians, hopelessly confounding the effects of the vitamin C. In response to these criticisms, Cameron and Pauling published a second study, noting that the same physicians had been involved with both sets of patients, and that the second control group matched the treatment group in all important respects, including stage of illness. The results for the second study were similar to those for the first, which seemed to offer a decisive answer to critics.[4]

Nevertheless, subsequent random-assignment, double-blind studies conducted by Mayo Clinic failed to replicate Pauling and Cameron's findings.[5] Pauling offered several reasons for this, including dosages that were too low, treatment regimens that were too short, and a patient population already ravaged by the effects of radiation and chemotherapy. While such criticisms sound like the standard litany from alternative medicine, the full gamut of evidence has persuaded much of the medical community that vitamin C helps prevent cancer, although the jury is still out about whether it has any benefit in cancer treatment. In September 1990, the National Institutes of Health sponsored a symposium to review the evidence regarding vitamin C, concluding that it does produce a protective effect.[6]

The change in attitude toward vitamin C and other nutritional supplements has been driven, in part, by a growing appreciation for antioxidants, which protect human cells from the damage caused by free radicals produced during the process of oxidation. A free radical is a molecule with an unpaired electron. Unstable and highly reactive, the molecule seeks to capture an electron that will stabilize it. By capturing electrons from nearby molecules, free radicals convert other molecules to free radicals, thereby initiating a destructive chain reaction. This process results in DNA damage, which leads to genetic mutation. Antioxidants reduce this damage by providing an alternative source of free electrons, helping to protect the DNA in normal cells. In addition to vitamin C, vitamins A and E are believed to be antioxidants, with vitamin E having the most potent antioxidant properties.

Free radicals have changed the way we think about many diseases, including cancer, heart disease, arthrosclerosis, cataracts, and arthritis. Some scientists believe that aging itself is primarily due to the cumulative effects of oxidation, which is inherent in the metabolic process required to sustain life. For example, the level of free radicals increases with vigorous exercise, when the metabolic rate is highest. Conversely, animal studies show that life span increases when the diet includes about 50 percent of normal caloric intake, which presumably correlates with a reduced rate of metabolism. Both findings suggest that life should be extended when free radicals are neutralized by antioxidants.

The concept of free radicals is critical to understanding many different aspects of medicine and physiology. For the reader conversant with the technical language of biochemistry, I recommend a chapter titled "Oxidant Stress and Host Oxidant Defense Mechanisms," by Ogino, Packer, and Traber, in the book *Nutritional Oncology.*[7] A less technical book is *The Antioxidant Miracle* by Packer and Colman.[8] Dr. Lester Packer, currently at the University of California, Berkeley, has been a leading investigator of antioxidants for many years. One of his most important contributions has been a reconceptualization of antioxidants: we should think of them not as operating independently, resulting in a summation of their effects, but as a network, where some antioxidants sustain the effects of others. For example, vitamin C may rejuvenate vitamin E after it has captured free radicals, allowing vitamin E to capture more free radicals. Similar functions are served by lipoic acid, selenium, and coenzyme Q_{10}, not only with respect to vitamin E, but also for glutathione, which Packer considers the most important antioxidant in the cell. Glutathione neutralizes free radicals, switches on the enzymes that repair DNA, and regulates the genes involved in arthritis, lupus, and other autoimmune diseases. Glutathione is produced by the body, but levels vary. Cancer patients typically have a reduced level. Increasing the level of glutathione is best accomplished by taking lipoic acid, one of its metabolic precursors.

The concept of an antioxidant network provides a different perspective on clinical trials that have tested antioxidants in isolation. In addition to Mayo Clinic's vitamin C trials, which failed to show any benefit, trials with beta-carotene, the precursor of vitamin A, also produced negative outcomes. In fact, two separate studies involving smokers reported that beta-carotene increased the incidence of lung cancer by 15 to 25 percent. This not only suggests that mega-dosages of vitamins may be harmful, it supports the conservative daily dosages recommended by nutritional and governmental agencies. But these conclusions are unwarranted, given that vitamin A may be effective if other elements of the network are present. In the absence of other critical antioxidants, high dosages of some vitamins may be pro-oxidant, especially when there is a great deal of oxidative stress in the environment (as is the case with smokers).

Epidemiological evidence suggests that eating fresh fruits and vegetables, which are rich in antioxidants, will reduce the risk of cancer. A number of studies tracking the consumption of fruits and vegetables have shown that people in the top quartile have a 50 percent lower incidence of cancer than those in the bottom quartile. This is why government agencies recommend at least five servings of fresh fruits and vegetables each day. It is uncertain, however, that antioxidants are responsible for these positive effects. Fruits and vegetables contain many other chemicals that have potent benefits. Moreover, people who adhere to a healthy diet often lead a healthy lifestyle in general: they tend to exercise more, avoid obesity, and refrain from smoking, all of which will help prevent cancer. While most epidemiological studies attempt to factor out these characteristics, it is impossible to do so completely; therefore, the validity of theories explaining the effects of fruits and vegetables remains uncertain.

It is entirely possible that some antioxidants play a role in preventing cancer but have no effect as a cancer treatment. This distinction was supported by a large, randomized clinical trial conducted in Finland.[9] The study evaluated the incidence of lung and prostate cancer for four groups of male smokers: those given a placebo, those receiving alpha-tocopherol (the most common form of vitamin E), those receiving beta-carotene, and those receiving both alpha-tocopherol and beta-carotene. Compared to the placebo, alpha-tocopherol reduced the incidence of prostate cancer by 32 percent and mortality from prostate cancer by 41 percent. It had no effect on lung cancer. Beta-carotene, on the other hand, produced a 23 percent higher incidence of prostate cancer (a result consistent with its effects on lung cancer) and a 15 percent higher mortality rate. Once prostate or lung cancer was diagnosed, neither vitamin had any effect on survival time.

Oncologists often advise patients to forego antioxidant supplements while undergoing cancer treatment. They argue that antioxidants undermine one of the mechanisms by which radiation and chemotherapy work, which is to increase the number of free radicals to a level that is fatal to cancer cells. This level is also damaging to normal cells, but these are assumed to have efficient DNA-repair mechanisms.

Proponents of alternative medicine, on the other hand, emphasize the need to protect normal cells. They claim that patients who receive antioxidants during treatment are healthier and have a better prognosis. Oncologists reply that nutritional support may make patients feel better, but this is deceptive, because antioxidants create the same effect as a lower dosage of radiation or chemotherapy.

To date, neither side of this argument has provided any clinical data that bear strongly on the issue; however, *American Journal of Clinical Nutrition* published a series of papers to highlight the debate. Those in favor of combining antioxidants with conventional cancer treatment[10] argued that it is essential to distinguish between different kinds of antioxidants. Some antioxidants seem to protect normal cells from the damaging effects of radiation and chemotherapy. Others inhibit various growth signaling channels that underlie many types of cancer. Still others activate genes for cell differentiation as well as the P53 tumor suppressor gene, which is critical for detecting genetic mutations. Proponents further argued that combining antioxidants often is more effective than using them individually. They cited several laboratory studies in which single antioxidants had no effect on cancer growth in cell cultures, while combinations almost completely inhibited the growth of cancer cells. They also described studies in which the combination of antioxidants and chemotherapy was much more effective than chemotherapy alone, including a nonrandomized clinical trial where patients with small cell lung cancer were treated with antioxidants in addition to the usual radiation and chemotherapy, which seemed to improve survival time relative to historical controls.[11]

Opponents to using antioxidants during radiation and chemotherapy[12] argued that free radicals play an important role in causing cancer cells to undergo apoptosis (programmed cell death). They described studies in which vitamin E decreased the cell death caused by cisplatin (one of the most common chemotherapy agents). They also cited a study[13] in which mice with implanted brain tumors were fed a diet either depleted of antioxidants or enriched with antioxidants. Tumor growth was substantially less for the depleted diet, while the rate of apoptosis was increased.

Except for the uncontrolled lung cancer study, I have been unable to find any clinical data that are clearly relevant to the debate. A number of clinical trials, however, have used combinations of nutrients, some of which were antioxidants. One small trial reported that nutritional supplements prolonged survival time for patients with non-small cell lung cancer. Patients receiving the standard treatment also consumed a freeze-dried soup containing selected vegetables. Patients who declined were treated as the control group. (This means that the trial did not involve random assignment.) The difference between the two groups was dramatic: those who declined the supplement had a median survival time of less than four months, while those receiving the supplement had a median survival of more than fifteen months. There was almost no overlap in the distribution of outcomes between the two groups.[14] A follow-up study[15] showed even longer survival times and included a laboratory experiment in which mice were fed a diet consisting of the soup ingredients. Tumor growth in the mice was inhibited by 50 to 75 percent.

The exact formula for the soup is not described, but it included cruciferous vegetables (such as broccoli and brussels sprouts), soybeans, shiitake mushrooms, mung beans, red dates, scallions, garlic, lentils, leaks, hawthorn fruit, onions, ginseng, angelica root, licorice, dandelion root, senega root, ginger, olives, sesame seeds, and parsley. These ingredients were chosen for their lack of toxicity and for their performance in anticancer laboratory studies. (Some of these ingredients, such as licorice root, also are used in SPES, the prostate cancer treatment described in chapter 12.) The diversity of ingredients precludes any analysis of which components were most effective. Nevertheless, the sizeable difference in outcomes makes this trial provocative, the lack of random assignment notwithstanding.

In a randomized trial reported at the 1999 annual meeting of the American Association for Cancer Research, supplements were used to treat localized prostate cancer.[16] Twenty men were scheduled to undergo surgical removal of their prostate. For three weeks prior to surgery, participants received either 15 mg of lycopene twice daily, or no intervention. (Lycopene, a form of vitamin A, is found in many red vegetables, especially tomatoes. Laboratory research indicates that it is perhaps the strongest antioxidant of the various forms of vitamin A.) When the prostate glands were analyzed following surgery, the lycopene group showed lower PSA counts as well as smaller tumors that were more likely to be confined to the prostate. While this small trial provides no information about lycopene's effect on survival, it does indicate that lycopene inhibits malignancy, at least temporarily.

Most of the research on antioxidants is in the beginning stages, so it is difficult to judge the efficacy of these nutritional supplements. To date, results have been provocative, giving credibility to proponents of alternative medicine who have advocated vitamin supplements for many years.

Supplements with Strong Evidence of Efficacy

MELATONIN

Melatonin, a hormone secreted by the pineal gland, regulates the diurnal and seasonal rhythms of the body.[17] Clinically it is used as an artificial method for resetting the biological clock, especially in travelers with jet lag and workers with irregular hours. Some experts believe that aging pineal glands secrete less melatonin, causing irregular sleep patterns in the elderly. In addition, melatonin has shown various effects on the immune system.

Several studies have failed to support claims about melatonin's effects on jet lag and irregular work schedules. Studies have also suggested that melatonin levels do not decrease as we age, therefore supplements may not help to regulate sleep patterns in the elderly. I have had considerable experience with melatonin, including reports from others who have used it, and I doubt that these criticisms are correct. I have seen too many cases where its effects have been quite potent, sometimes excessively so (some people report feeling groggy after they awake in the morning). Only time will tell how such informal observations will be reconciled with the clinical trial results.

Melatonin is available in any drugstore in the United States and in most grocery stores. In Europe, where it is considered a neurohormone with unknown toxicity, it is available only by prescription. Although extremely high dosages have demonstrated no toxicity in standard tests, some investigators are concerned that deleterious effects may still occur, including damage to the reproductive system or changes in the sensitivity of melatonin receptors. Such speculation persists because we know very little about how melatonin works.

Effects of melatonin on the immune system have, in fact, been identified.[18] It functions as an antioxidant scavenger for hydroxyl radicals, thereby preventing DNA damage; induces various cytokines by the T cells, including TNF-alpha, interleukin-1, interleukin-2, and gamma-interferon; and provides an antigen-independent influence on natural killer cell activity. All of these improve the body's ability to cope with foreign proteins. There is also evidence that melatonin has direct cytotoxic effects on some types of cancer cells, especially melanoma and prostate cancer, although the mechanism by which this occurs is unknown.

Most of the research on melatonin as a cancer treatment has been conducted in Italy. When I discovered these studies, which included a randomized clinical trial for glioblastoma patients, I was surprised that American oncologists had no interest in the findings. Whether this reflects a bias against foreign research or skepticism about alternative medicine is unclear. Perhaps American oncology rejects melatonin because it is a component of the controversial Revici cancer protocol, which American oncologists believe has been discredited.

There is considerable evidence supporting melatonin as an anti-cancer agent. It has been used in combination with low dosages of interleukin-2, a treatment regimen regarded at least as effective as high dosages of interleukin-2 but without the associated toxicity. Also, research suggests that melatonin helps alleviate the toxic effects of chemotherapy, especially with respect to platelet count.

Phase-II clinical trials have studied melatonin in cancer patients who failed their initial treatment. These included metastatic prostate patients after androgen-suppression therapy failed, metastatic breast cancer patients who failed tamoxifen therapy, and various patients with colorectal, pancreatic, uterine, liver, ovarian, and lung cancer. A number of these patients, who were rapidly deteriorating prior to melatonin treatment, had their disease stabilize, and a few had their tumors recede. Such data do not, of course, prove that melatonin is an effective treatment for cancer. Cancer progression can be highly variable, and melatonin's effects need to be quantified before any evaluation is made.

Randomized clinical trials have compared patients receiving melatonin plus the standard treatment with patients receiving only the standard treatment. These have included glioblastoma patients who failed radiation therapy,[19] non-small cell lung cancer patients who failed cisplatin chemotherapy,[20] node-relapsed melanoma patients,[21] and colorectal cancer patients who failed 5-fluorouracil chemotherapy.[22] In every case, patients receiving melatonin had, on average, a longer survival time than those not receiving it. This does not mean that melatonin provided a cure, only that it improved the duration of life.

In yet another study, patients with non-small cell lung cancer received cisplatin, etoposide, and melatonin as a first-line treatment.[23] For those receiving etoposide and cisplatin without melatonin, the one-year survival rate was approximately 19 percent; for patients receiving all three agents, the survival rate was 44 percent. In addition, melatonin appeared to increase quality of life.

In a more extensive randomized clinical trial, patients with advanced metastatic cancer were randomly assigned to receive chemotherapy alone or with 20 mg/day of melatonin.[24] Objective tumor regressions (including six complete regressions) occurred in 42 of 124 patients who received the melatonin, but in only 19 of the 126 control patients (with no complete regressions). In the melatonin group, 63 patients were alive after one year, compared to 29 in the control group. Such results are an improvement over those produced by conventional treatments, especially considering that the trial patients were in an advanced state of disease.

Although melatonin shows clear evidence of efficacy, it seems to be completely ignored by American medicine. Perhaps there is no better example of the need for patients to conduct their own search for information.

PSK, LENTINAN, AND OTHER POLYSACCHARIDES

Several Asian countries use mushroom extracts, classified as biological response modifiers, in their cancer protocols. Most of the research on these extracts has been conducted in Japan and only sporadically reported in American journals. Studies have been so impressive that a half-dozen of these extracts are now widely used by Japanese cancer patients. In fact, they are covered by the Japanese national health insurance as part of the standard treatment for several types of cancer.

The most widely investigated extracts are PSK (polysaccharide krestin), from the mushroom *Coriolus versicolor,* and lentinan, from shi-itake mushrooms. PSK can be taken orally while lentinan is given by injection. As yet, there is no clear indication that one is better than the other. Both are believed to enhance the immune system through gamma-interferon production, interleukin-2 production, and increased T cell activity.[25] Moreover, in vitro studies have shown cytotoxic effects through the inhibition of matrix-degrading enzymes, which underlie tumor invasion of adjacent tissue, and the inhibition of angiogenesis.[26]

These polysaccharides also have been shown to increase resistance to bacterial, viral, and parasitic infections in AIDS patients.[27] Neither extract has shown any toxicity.

PSK and lentinan may prolong life for patients with advanced and recurrent stomach cancer, colorectal cancer, breast cancer, leukemia, and non-small cell lung cancer. In one representative study involving non-small cell lung cancer, stage-I patients receiving 3 g/day PSK had a five-year survival rate of 39 percent, compared to 17 percent for patients not receiving PSK. For stage-III patients, the five-year survival rate was 26 percent with PSK and 8 percent without. Both differences were statistically significant.[28] Studies involving colon cancer and stomach cancer have also shown that PSK improves survival rates.

Another study tested PSK as a treatment for glioma in combination with ACNU (a chemical cousin of BCNU) and vincristine.[29] The survival rate for glioblastoma patients was 56 percent after one year and 37 percent after two years. Because there was no control group, the exact effect of PSK was unclear; however, the two-year survival rate was much greater than the rate typically produced by traditional treatments.

Unfortunately, neither PSK nor lentinan is easy to obtain in this country. A small vendor in Eugene, Oregon, sells a month's supply of PSK for $125.[30] Lentinan, however, requires an injectable solution and is not available in the United States. Health-food stores offer oral extracts of maitake, shiitake, reishi, and other mushrooms having polysaccharide similar to lentinan. Of these, maitake D-fraction (a liquid extract of the whole mushroom) may be the most effective.[31] In one experiment, 93 percent of mice injected with a known carcinogen developed tumors within forty-five days, compared to only 30 percent of injected mice that were fed maitake D-fraction. In a second controlled experiment, maitake D-fraction inhibited 90 percent of breast tumor growth. A third experiment combined the extract with chemotherapy, inhibiting 87 percent of metastatic tumors from injected liver cancer cells. (Chemotherapy alone inhibited only 50 percent.) The authors of these studies noted that comparable experiments with lentinan produced much smaller effects.

The active ingredient in these mushroom extracts is believed to be a molecule called beta glucan. Nutriceutical producers have begun to market this agent, which also comes from bovine cartilage, complex grain proteins, and other sources. There is no easy way to evaluate the relative effectiveness of the different products.

Despite extensive clinical literature in Japan that shows mushroom extracts are a valuable adjunct to conventional cancer treatment, American oncologists have generally ignored them, and most patients never learn of their existence.

GLA AND OTHER ESSENTIAL POLYUNSATURATED FATTY ACIDS

I discovered gamma-linolenic acid (GLA) as a potential glioblastoma treatment after reading an Indian study that showed major tumor regression when GLA was infused directly into the tumor cavity. As I delved more deeply into fatty acids and their effects on cancer, I realized that this was perhaps the most complex topic in the biochemistry of oncology.

There are several kinds of fatty acids, but only polyunsaturated fats appear relevant to cancer prevention or treatment. Monounsaturated fats, such as olive oil, and saturated fats, such as those found in meat, apparently play little role in cancer, though the latter has been linked to cardiovascular disease.

Polyunsaturated fatty acids are divided into two general classes: omega-3s and omega-6s. The omega-3s include alpha-linoleic acid (found in flax seed oil and perilla oil) and its major derivatives, eicosapentenoic (EPA) and docosahexaenoic (DHA) acids (most abundant in fish oil). The basic omega-6 fatty acid is linoleic acid, found in corn oil and soybean oil. Linoleic acid metabolizes into GLA, which then breaks down into either dihomo-gamma-linoleic acid or arachidonic acid. Each of these categories includes numerous subvarieties with different biochemical properties.

The general consensus, which is by no means unanimous, is that omega-3s help prevent cancer while omega-6s promote it. Accordingly, taking fish oil supplements and avoiding corn oil should reduce the risk of cancer, a conclusion based mainly on studies of breast and prostate cancer in rodents. In theory, different fatty acids promote different prostaglandins, critical components of the inflammatory process by which the immune system deals with foreign proteins. Type-II prostaglandins, which are stimulated by arachidonic acid, are believed to produce powerful inflammatory reactions. Type-I prostaglandins, which are stimulated by omega-3 fatty acids, modulate this inflammatory effect.

Underlying this thinking is the assumption that an overstimulated inflammatory process promotes cancer. There is evidence that this is true, at least for some forms of cancer. For example, the risk of colon cancer is reduced through the regular use of anti-inflammatory drugs, such as ibuprofen.[32] This is somewhat counterintuitive, because one might expect agents that strengthen the inflammatory process to have beneficial effects. If the immune system vigorously attacks any foreign protein, should it not be more likely to eradicate the genetic mutations that cause cancer? But intuition is of little use in understanding something as complicated as the immune system.

It is possible that the inflammatory process plays opposite roles in cancer prevention and cancer treatment. Any conclusions about different fatty acids depend on the type of cancer for which they are assessed. Generalizations are further limited by the fact that GLA, an omega-6 fatty acid, has anti-inflammatory properties. Studies have shown that GLA may be an effective treatment for rheumatoid arthritis, an autoimmune disease.[33] This seems paradoxical, since omega-6s are believed to have an inflammatory effect.

Given the complex interactions that seem to occur between fatty acids, there is little basis for predicting how they should function as therapeutic agents. We must therefore examine the actual data, rather

SURVIVING "TERMINAL" CANCER

than draw inferences from supposed mechanisms of action. A comprehensive review of the effects of fatty acids was published in 1998,[34] as the result of an international symposium. According to these sources, there is no doubt that essential fatty acids have enormous potential in cancer treatment.

In the laboratory, cancer cell lines have shown vulnerability to several fatty acids, especially GLA and EPA. There may be several mechanisms involved in creating this cytotoxicity. The best documented is the metabolization of fatty acids by cancer cells, which creates a high level of free radicals that are lethal to malignant cells. This conclusion is based on the fact that antioxidants (such as vitamin E) reduce cytotoxicity while pro-oxidants (such as iron) increase it. Other possible mechanisms include the inhibition of angiogenesis, the up-regulation of the P53 tumor suppressor gene, the enhanced expression of cell-cell adhesion molecules (which help prevent cancer cells from spreading), and the inhibition of protein kinase C (a major growth signaling channel). Fatty acids are also known to change the structure of cell membranes, which is believed to increase the effectiveness of both chemotherapy and radiation. At the same time, they have been shown to protect normal cells from radiation damage.

Until recently, the only fatty acid used in clinical settings was gamma-linolenic acid. Earlier I described an Indian trial where glioma patients received infusions of GLA directly into the tumor cavity.[35] Of the fifteen patients treated, most had tumor regressions, and twelve of the fifteen were alive at the time the report was published. The three who died were quite elderly. Because of the dramatic results, I contacted the lead author of the publication to determine if anyone outside of India was using the procedure. He referred me to a neurosurgeon in Wales who had used it, but without the degree of success reported in India. Although the Welsh procedure did show considerable efficacy, the neurosurgeon was concerned that the alcohol needed to dissolve the GLA may have a harmful effect on the brain. (Like other fats, GLA is not water soluble.)

A more recent clinical trial compared the use of oral GLA plus tamoxifen vs. tamoxifen alone for advanced breast cancer patients.[36] Three months after the initiation of treatment, 5 percent of patients receiving the combination showed a complete response (compared to zero patients receiving only tamoxifen), and 37 percent had partial regression (compared to 13 percent in the tamoxifen group). All but a small fraction of the remaining subjects in both groups had stable disease.

Another GLA trial is in progress at Adderbrooke Hospital in Cambridge, England, where GLA is being given to patients with pancreatic cancer, glioblastoma's principal rival as the most deadly type of cancer. In this trial, GLA is combined with a lithium salt to make it water soluble, then administered intravenously. Phase-I results seem promising, with survival times exceeding those typically produced by conventional means.[37]

Another trial compared the effects of fish oil supplements vs. a placebo in treating several different types of advanced cancer.[38] Thirty patients who were malnourished from cachexia were randomly assigned to receive either a placebo or a combination of 18 g/day fish oil and 200 mg/day vitamin E. An additional thirty patients who were not suffering from malnutrition received a similar random assignment. In both groups, the combination of fish oil and vitamin E significantly increased median survival time (210 days vs. 110 days for the malnourished patients, and 500 days vs. 350 days for the nourished patients).

In the United States, the only sources of GLA are supplements made from various seed oils. The most common are primrose oil, borage seed oil, and black currant seed oil, which are available in any health-food store. Primrose oil contains a 10 percent concentration of GLA. Borage seed oil has about twice that concentration, approximately 20 to 25 percent. It is uncertain that taking these supplements will provide enough GLA to have a significant anticancer effect; however, the breast cancer trial described above suggests that oral ingestion does, indeed, provide a clinical benefit.

None of these essential fatty acids have shown toxicity at any dosage studied. Thus, if a cancer patient can tolerate enough borage seed capsules to reach the level of 3 g/day of GLA, as well as the financial cost, it may be worth a try, especially in combination with chemotherapy. Chemotherapy and GLA appear to have similar cytotoxic mechanisms, and GLA seems to enhance the permeability of cell membranes, allowing chemotherapy to enter more easily. Furthermore, recent evidence suggests that GLA has antiangiogenic effects and may be synergistic with tamoxifen.

In light of recent evidence, conjugated linoleic acid (CLA), an isomer form of linoleic acid found in red meat and cheese, should also be considered. In laboratory studies with rats and mice, CLA has shown strong anticancer properties, notably against breast and prostate tumors, colorectal and stomach cancer, and melanoma.[39] Concentrations of CLA that had cytotoxic effects in the laboratory are easily achieved through diet or supplements. For example, eating cheddar cheese appears to produce therapeutic concentrations of CLA. So does taking commercial supplements, which are produced by a special isomerization treatment of sunflower oil.

CLA has remarkable properties in addition to its anticancer effects. These include the ability to act as an insulin sensitizer, lowering insulin resistance and insulin levels. (This should be of special interest to people with type-II diabetes.) It also lowers the percentage of body weight composed of fat, perhaps by increasing metabolic rate. Despite its benefits—and its lack of toxicity, even at very high dosages—no clinical studies of CLA have been reported.

GENISTEIN

Genistein is an isoflavone found in soy products. Epidemiological data suggests a correlation between the consumption of soy and a lower incidence of cancer, although this finding may have been confounded by other dietary factors. For example, cultures that consume large amounts of soy often consume green tea as well—another agent suspected of having anticancer properties. These studies, however, are supported by laboratory research that identified anticancer effects. Much of this research was presented in 1996 at an international meeting on the health benefits of soy; the proceedings were published in 1998. Of all the ingredients discussed, genistein appears to be the most important for cancer treatment.[40]

I first learned of genistein while searching for information about low-intensity brachytherapy. I found only three places in the United States that used low-intensity implants, including the University of Vermont. When I called the principal investigator, he explained that they had used the procedure with only a few patients and without notable success. He then expressed excitement about his recent research on genistein. His laboratory studies indicated that genistein inhibited the migration of glioblastoma cells from the original tumor site, and that the required dosage could be achieved simply by consuming more soy products. He also indicated that considerably higher concentrations of genistein had a cytotoxic effect.[41]

At that time, there were only a few soy extracts on the market, and these had relatively low concentrations of genistein. Two years later, The Life Extension Foundation introduced a supplement with a genistein concentration ten times greater than anything else available, and I have taken it ever since. Up until then, I did my best to increase my soy intake with soy burgers, soy milk, soy nuts, and so forth, along with supplements containing the highest genistein concentrations available. This became a tiresome feeding regimen that required some willpower to sustain.

I began researching the basis of genistein's effects to determine if it was worth the trouble. This has been an ongoing effort, as more and more studies are recognizing that genistein is a powerful anticancer agent. In one experiment, mice were fed different concentrations of genistein, then injected with melanoma cells known to cause lung metastases. Depending on the amount of genistein added to the diet, the number of tumors were reduced by approximately 50 to 75 percent.[42] An earlier study reported an even larger inhibitory effect when whole soy extracts were added to the diet rather than genistein alone. Numerous laboratory studies have produced comparable results.

Apparently, most of genistein's anticancer properties result from its ability to block the epidermal growth factor receptors on the cell membrane. These receptors provide a signal that allows cells to divide. Cancer cells have a huge number of these receptors, causing the cells to divide wildly. Blocking these receptors cause cancer cells to either differentiate into normal cells or die. With a growing recognition of the importance of these receptors, at least a half-dozen drug companies are developing their own inhibitory agents, usually in the form of monoclonal antibodies. In addition to blocking the epidermal growth factor receptors, genistein seems to inhibit protein kinase C, which appears to be a critical signal that causes malignant growth in gliomas. Because tamoxifen also inhibits protein kinase C, there is reason to believe that a combination of genistein and tamoxifen might be especially effective.[43] Finally, there is increasing evidence that genistein prevents angiogenesis.[44]

Human clinical trials using genistein as a cancer treatment are currently in progress. Genistein was isolated in 1987, and only now is there enough laboratory evidence to inspire clinical development. Whether such development will occur remains to be seen. Pharmaceutical companies have little incentive because genistein is not patentable. Development will likely require government intervention, which has not been forthcoming.

Potential Supplements for Cancer Treatment and Prevention

In addition to melatonin, PSK, GLA, and genistein, another half-dozen dietary supplements have been shown to help prevent cancer or regress existing tumors. Some of these are being studied in phase-I clinical trials. Though the evidence for their effects is still fragmentary, at least some of these agents will become players in nutritional-based cancer treatment programs, which are only a few years away. The government will need to develop these programs, since they clearly are not in the interests of pharmaceutical companies. The ingredients are too easily obtained to be patentable, and they will directly compete with the pharmaceutical companies' cancer drugs.

SELENIUM

The potency of this trace element was discovered almost by accident in a randomized, placebo-controlled clinical trial. Selenium, commonly found in onions and garlic, was being tested as a preventative agent for skin cancer. While it had no effect on the incidence of skin cancer, it had a substantial effect on the incidence of other types of cancer, including lung, colorectal, and prostate. The most dramatic results occurred in prostate cancer—its incidence was reduced by 63 percent among those receiving selenium.[45]

Laboratory research suggests that selenium should also be effective in treating cancer. It has been shown to inhibit tumor growth in vitro, and selenium supplements have inhibited pulmonary metastases when melanoma cells were injected into mice. Recent studies also suggest that selenium strongly inhibits the growth of glioma cells cultured in the laboratory.[46]

GREEN TEA

In both China and Japan, green tea has been consumed for 5,000 years because of its supposed medicinal properties. Its primary anticancer ingredients are believed to be polyphenolic catechins, the most prominent of which is epigallocatechin-3-gallate (EGCG).

Green tea has produced anticancer effects in rats and mice, both for implanted and carcinogen-induced tumors.[47] Furthermore, the National Institutes of Health has singled out green tea as the most promising alternative agent warranting further research. As yet, there are no available data from clinical trials that allow us to evaluate the usefulness of green tea; however, given that there is no downside to its use, green tea could be added to any cancer treatment program.

LIMONENE

Limonene is a monoterpene, a constituent of the essential oils found in citrus fruits and other plants. Derived from the skin of citrus, it is not unlike the lemon oil used for conditioning wooden furniture.

In laboratory studies, limonene, along with its derivative, perillyl alcohol, has shown anticancer effects against liver, breast, lung, and pancreatic cancer, as well as leukemia and neuroblastoma. It is currently being studied in human clinical trials. Like other dietary supplements, it may work best in combination with other agents. One human clinical trial has combined limonene with lovastatin, a common drug used to lower cholesterol. Early results indicate that some subjects have had prolonged periods of remission.[48]

QUERCETIN

Quercetin is one of the flavonoids found in plants. Its most common sources are onions and apples. Like genistein, quercetin appears to inhibit tyrosine kinase activity, and laboratory studies combining quercetin and genistein have shown a synergistic effect for both ovarian and breast cancer cells.[49] It currently is under investigation in phase-I clinical trials.

WHEY PROTEIN

Whey protein is marketed as the highest quality of any form of protein, mainly for those engaged in vigorous athletic activity. In several laboratory studies, rats and mice were fed a whey protein diet while given cancer-inducing chemicals. These animals developed far fewer tumors than rodents that did not receive a whey protein diet, and the tumors that did develop were much smaller.

An anticancer effect is believed to occur because whey protein depletes the glutathione levels of cancer cells but not of normal cells. Glutathione enables a rapid repair of damage caused by chemotherapy; elevated levels may be one reason that cancer cells are resistant to chemotherapy treatment. Reducing the glutathione levels should prevent such repair and make chemotherapy more effective.

One small clinical trial used a whey protein product called Immunocal. Seven patients with different kinds of advanced cancer were fed 30 g/day of whey protein for six months. Two patients had tumor regression, while two others showed tumor stabilization.[50] No clinical trials combining whey protein with chemotherapy have yet been reported.

BROCCOLI SPROUTS

My favorite cancer treatment, newly arrived on the scene, is broccoli sprouts. George Bush the senior notwithstanding, broccoli sprouts are a tasty addition to salads, and there exists an inverse relation between cancer risk and the consumption of brassica vegetables (broccoli, cauliflower, brussels sprouts, and cabbage). The prevailing theory is that their anticancer effects are due to a substance called sulforaphane.[51] Three-to-four-day-old sprouts contain 10 to 100 times the amount of sulforaphane found in the full-grown vegetables. To test whether oral ingestion of these sprouts have an anticancer effect, dried broccoli sprouts were fed to rats with induced cancers, resulting in considerable tumor regression.[52]

Other potential anticancer supplements have been identified, including coenzyme Q_{10}, DHEA, phytic acid (found in many whole grains), and curcumin (found in turmeric). As the identification of anticancer foods becomes a more intensive enterprise, it is only a matter of time before more ingredients are isolated and purified for investigation.

A test for the nation's cancer agenda is how the next stage of development will be managed. Given that most food ingredients are commonly available, pharmaceutical companies are unlikely to have the economic motivation to research these substances. And because of the extraordinary costs inherent in the FDA-controlled regulatory process, advocates of alternative medicine will be unable to sponsor their development. Will the government fill the breach? I have strong doubts that it will. Fortunately, the alternative medicine community will continue to popularize the value of these supplements. Otherwise, cancer patients would not learn about easily obtainable agents that may improve their prognoses.

ENDNOTES

1. For information about The Life Extension Foundation, go to www.lef.org, call 1-800-820-3251, or write to The Life Extension Foundation, P.O. Box 229120, Hollywood, Florida, 33022.

2. It is bad enough that a government agency has engaged in the erroneous characterization of a pharmaceutical product. Much more serious is that this agency has the power to prosecute individuals who import drugs that are approved in Europe but not in the United States. At issue is the right of individual Americans to obtain medications, regardless of FDA approval, when solid evidence indicates that the drugs may provide a benefit.

3. Cameron, E., and Pauling, L. Supplemental ascorbate in the supportive treatment of cancer: prolongation of survival times in terminal human cancer. *Proceedings of the National Academy of Sciences.* 1976;73(10):3685-3689.

4. Cameron, E., and Pauling, L. Supplemental ascorbate in the supportive treatment of cancer: reevaluation of prolongation of survival times in terminal human cancer. *Proceedings of the National Academy of Sciences.* 1978;75(9):4538-4542.

5. Creagan, E. T., et al. Failure of high-dose vitamin C (ascorbic acid) therapy to benefit patients with advanced cancer: a controlled trial. *New England Journal of Medicine.* 1979;301(13):687-690.

6. Ascorbic acid: biologic functions and relation to cancer. Proceedings of a conference held at the National Institutes of Health, Bethesda, Maryland. 1990 Sept 10-12. *American Journal of Clinical Nutrition.* 1991;54(suppl 6):1113S-1327S.

7. Ogino, T., et al. Oxidant stress and host oxidant defense mechanisms. In: Heber, D., Blackburn, G., and Go, V., eds. *Nutritional Oncology.* San Diego: Academic Press; 1999:253-275.

8. Packer, L., and Colman, C. *The Antioxidant Miracle.* New York: John Wiley and Sons; 1999.

9. The Alpha-Tocopherol/Beta-Carotene Cancer Prevention Study Group: the effect of vitamin E and beta-carotene on the incidence of lung cancer and other cancer in male smokers. *New England Journal of Medicine.* 1994;330:1029-1035.

10. Prasad, K. N., et al. Scientific rationale for using high-dose multiple micronutrients as an adjunct to standard and experimental cancer therapies. *Journal of the American College of Nutrition.* 2001 Oct;(suppl 5):450S-463S.

11. Prasad, K. N., et al. High doses of multiple antioxidant vitamins: essential ingredients in improving the efficacy of standard cancer therapy. *Journal of the American College of Nutrition.* 1999 Feb;18(1):13-25.

12. Salganik, R. I. The benefits and hazards of antioxidants: controlling apoptosis and other protective mechanisms in cancer patients and the human population. *Journal of the American College of Nutrition.* 2001 Oct;20(suppl 5):464S-472S.

13. Salganik, R. I., et al. Dietary antioxidant depletion: enhancement of tumor apoptosis and inhibition of brain tumor growth in transgenic mice. *Carcinogenesis.* 2000 May;21(5):909-914.

14. Sun, A. S., et al. Phase-I/II study of stage-III and -IV non-small cell lung cancer patients taking a specific dietary supplement. *Nutrition and Cancer.* 1999;34(1)62-69.

15. Sun, A. S., et al. Pilot study of a specific dietary supplement in tumor-bearing mice and in stage-IIIB and -IV non-small cell lung cancer patients. *Nutrition and Cancer.* 2001;39(1):85-95.

16. Kucuk, O., et al. Phase-II randomized clinical trial of lycopene supplementation before radical prostatectomy. *Cancer Epidemiology, Biomarkers and Prevention.* 2001;10(8):861-868.

17. Descartes considered the pineal gland to be the site of interaction between mind and body, allowing the mind access to instruct the body on how to behave. His rationale was that the pineal gland was the only brain structure that he could identify that was not bilateral. For years, neurologists had no idea what its function was and regarded it as akin to the appendix—a relic of evolution that served no adaptive purpose. We now know that the pineal gland secretes melatonin and a variety of other hormones.

18. Neri, B., et al. Melatonin as biological response modifier in cancer patients. *Anticancer Research.* 1998;18(2B):1329-1332.

19. Lissoni, P., et al. Increased survival time in brain glioblastomas by a radioneuroendocrine strategy with radiotherapy plus melatonin compared to radiotherapy alone. *Oncology.* 1996;53(1):43-46.

20. Lissoni, P., et al. Randomized study with the pineal hormone melatonin versus supportive care alone in advanced nonsmall cell lung cancer resistant to a first-line chemotherapy containing cisplatin. *Oncology.* 1992;49(5)336-339.

21. Lissoni, P., et al. Adjuvant therapy with the pineal hormone melatonin in patients with lymph node relapse due to malignant growth. *Journal of Pineal Research.* 1996;21(4):239-242.

22. Barni, S., et al. A randomized study of low-dose subcutaneous interleukin-2 plus melatonin versus supportive care alone in metastatic colorectal cancer patients progressing under 5-fluorouracil and folates. *Oncology.* 1995;52(3):243-245.

23. Lissoni, P., et al. A randomized study of chemotherapy with cisplatin plus etoposide versus chemoendocrine therapy with cisplatin, etoposide, and the pineal hormone as a first-line treatment of advanced non-small cell lung cancer patients in a poor clinical state. *Journal of Pineal Research.* 1997;23(1):15-19.

24. See note 18.

25. Tsukagoshi, S., et al. Krestin (PSK). *Cancer Treatment Reviews.* 1984;11(2):131-155.

26. Kobayashi, H., et al. Antimetastatic effects of PSK (Krestin), a protein-bound polysaccharide obtained from Basidiomycetes: an overview. *Cancer Epidemiology, Biomarkers, and Prevention.* 1995;4(3):275-281.

27. Chihara, G. Recent progress in immunopharmacology and therapeutic effects of polysaccharides. *Developments in Biological Standardization.* 1992;77:191-197.

28. Hayakawa, K., et al. Effect of Krestin as adjuvant treatment following radical radiotherapy in non-small cell lung cancer patients. *Cancer Detection and Prevention.* 1997;21(1):71-77.

29. Kaneko, S., et al. Evaluation of radiation immunochemotherapy in the treatment of malignant glioma: combined use of ACNU, VCR and PSK. *Hokkaido Journal of Medical Science.* 1983;58:622-630.

30. JHS Natural Products, P.O. Box 50398, Eugene, Oregon, 97405; 1-542-341-1396.

31. Nanba, H., and Kubo, K. Effect of maitake D-fraction on cancer prevention. *Annals of New York Academy of Sciences.* 1997;833:204-207.

32. DuBois, A. N. Nonsteroidal anti-inflammatory drugs and prevention of colorectal cancer. *Current Gastroenterology Reports.* 1999 Oct;1(5):441-448.

33. Zurier, R. B., et al. Gamma-linolenic acid treatment of rheumatoid arthritis: a randomized placebo-controlled trial. *Arthritis and Rheumatism.* 1996;39(11):1808-1817.

34. Jiang, W. G., et al. Essential fatty acids: molecular and cellular basis of their anti-cancer action and clinical implications. *Critical Reviews in Oncology/Hematology.* 1998;27(3):179-209.

35. See chapter 3, note 9.

36. Kenny, F. S., et al. Gamma-linolenic acid with tamoxifen as primary therapy in breast cancer. *International Journal of Cancer.* 2000;85(5):643-648.

37. Fearoni, K. C. H., et al. An open-label phase-I/II escalation study of the treatment of pancreatic cancer using lithium gammalinolenate. *Anticancer Research.* 1996;16:867-874.

38. Gogos, C. A., et al. Dietary omega-3 polyunsaturated fatty acids plus vitamin E restore immunodeficiency and prolong survival for severely ill patients with generalized malignancy: a randomized control trial. *Cancer.* 1998;82(2):395-402.

39. Ip, C. Review of the effects of transfatty acids, oleic acid, n-3 polyunsaturated fatty acids, and conjugated linoleic acid on mammary carcinogenesis in animals. *American Journal of Clinical Nutrition.* 1997;66(suppl 6):1523S-1529S.

40. Second International Symposium on the Role of Soy in Preventing and Treating Chronic Disease, Brussels, Belgium, September 1996. Proceedings published in *American Journal of Clinical Nutrition.* 1998;68(suppl 6).

41. Penar, P. L., et al. Inhibition of epidermal growth factor receptor-associated tyrosine kinase blocks glioblastoma invasion of the brain. *Neurosurgery.* 1997;40(1):141-151.

42. Li, D., et al. Soybean isoflavones reduce experimental metastasis in mice. *Journal of Nutrition.* 1999;129(5):1075-1078.

43. Baltuch, G. H., and Yong, V. W. Signal transduction for proliferation of glioma cells in vitro occurs predominantly through a protein kinase C-mediated pathway. *Brain Research.* 1996;710(1-2):143-149.

44. Zhou, J. R., et al. Soybean phytochemicals inhibit the growth of transplantable prostate carcinoma and tumor angiogenesis in mice. *Journal of Nutrition.* 1999;129(9):1628-1635.

45. Clark, L. C., et al. Effects of selenium supplementation for cancer prevention in patients with carcinoma of the skin: a randomized controlled trial. Nutritional Prevention of Cancer Study Group. *Journal of the American Medical Association.* 1996;276(24):1957-1963.

46. Sundaram, N., et al. Selenium causes growth inhibition and apoptosis in human brain tumor cell lines. *Journal of Neuro-oncology.* 2000;46(2):125-133.

47. Kuroda, Y., and Hara, Y. Antimutagenic and anticarcinogenic activity of tea polyphenols. *Mutation Research.* 1999;436(1):69-97.

48. Vigushin, D. M., et al. Phase-I and pharmacokinetic study of D-limonene in patients with advanced cancer. Cancer Research Campaign Phase-I/II Clinical Trials Committee. *Cancer Chemotherapy and Pharmacology.* 1998;42(2):111-117.

49. Shen, F., and Weber, G. Synergistic action of quercetin and genistein in human ovarian carcinoma cells. *Oncology Research.* 1997;9(11-12):597-602.

50. Kennedy, R. S., et al. The use of a whey protein concentrate in the treatment of patients with metastatic carcinoma: a phase I-II clinical study. *Anticancer Research.* 1995;15(6B):2643-2649.

51. Verhoeven, D. T., et al. A review of mechanisms underlying anticarcinogenesis by brassica vegetables. *Chemico-Biological Interactions.* 1997;103(2):79-129.

52. Fahey, J. W., et al. Broccoli sprouts: an exceptionally rich source of inducers of enzymes that protect against chemical carcinogens. *Proceedings of the National Academy of Sciences.* 1997;94(19):10367-10372.

The Cutting Edge of Cancer Treatment

CHAPTER FOURTEEN

IN 1971, RICHARD NIXON DECLARED THE WAR ON CANCER, A NATIONAL mission having the same level of dedication as NASA's effort to put a man on the moon. Unfortunately, the War on Cancer has been notably less successful. Approximately 500,000 people in the United States die of cancer each year, and the rate of cancer death has risen steadily over the past twenty years. While part of this increase stems from a growing elderly population, which has a higher incidence of cancer, much of the increase is due to unknown causes. Some cancers, like melanoma, are influenced by known environmental hazards, while others, like lung cancer, are clearly affected by lifestyle choices. (Both the decrease in the male death rate and the increase in the female death rate are directly related to changes in smoking behavior.) But in general, we know little more about what causes cancer than we did when Nixon declared his War.

We are equally ignorant about how to cure this disease, although a few cancers, including Hodgkin's disease, childhood leukemia, and testicular cancer, now have successful treatments. Two decades ago, these were believed to carry a death sentence. Today, patients afflicted with these diseases are generally cured. Moreover, notable improvements in survival time have occurred for ovarian cancer and lymphoma. But such success stories are the exception. The five-year survival rate for most cancers has changed little since 1965, and the small improvements that have occurred are primarily due to earlier detection methods, such as the mammogram for breast cancer and the PSA test for prostate cancer. Chemotherapy, the primary weapon in cancer treatment, has not notably improved the prognosis for breast, lung, prostate, and colon cancers, which constitute the great majority of cancer cases.[1]

The War on Cancer has been conducted on a puny scale. Although Nixon's declaration resulted in a sizeable infusion of research funds, the amount has clearly been inadequate, as promising treatments have gone unexplored because of a lack of government funding. When compared to other government expenditures, the War on Cancer simply is not high on the nation's list of priorities. In fact, the current level of funding is considerably less than what the Department of Agriculture pays farmers to restrict the amount of food they produce in order to maintain price supports. This benefits ten million farmers at most, while raising food costs for the general population. In contrast, 40 percent of Americans will be diagnosed with cancer during their lifetime. If the American people knew how their money was being spent, such bizarre budgetary priorities would be unlikely to continue.

Advocates of alternative medicine argue that funds for cancer research have been badly spent and largely wasted. They contend that "slash, burn, and poison" continues to dominate cancer treatment not because it serves patients, but because it furthers the interests of the pharmaceutical and medical establishments. They therefore insist that greater emphasis be placed on eliminating environmental causes of cancer and boosting the immune systems of cancer patients.

SURVIVING "TERMINAL" CANCER

In terms of improving survival rates, this argument has considerable merit. Authoritative reviews estimate that cancer mortality would decline 70 percent if people changed their diet, eliminated tobacco products, reduced alcohol intake, increased physical exercise, and had routine exams for colorectal, prostate, and breast cancer. Of course, there are limits to how much a government can change the behavior of citizens in a free society. Human behavior is largely controlled by its immediate consequences. Inevitably, treatments for the effects of such bad choices as smoking and excessive sun exposure will always be an important priority. Such treatments are also necessary for the majority of cancers that have no clear etiology, including brain cancer.

I concur with proponents of alternative medicine who observe that the past twenty-five years of research have produced little success in terms of clinical outcome. On the other hand, scientific developments have been percolating under the surface of current cancer protocols, developments that will totally transform the future of cancer treatment. Since the discovery of DNA in the 1950s, our understanding of cell division and what goes wrong when cells become malignant has continuously increased. As a result, science has identified a number of targets for intervening in the process of malignant growth. We are on the edge of bringing this new knowledge into a clinical setting. How long it will take remains to be seen, especially given the bureaucratic impediments strewn along the path of development.

The following pages provide an overview of scientific advances that may transform cancer treatment. Some of these are in clinical trials and may be only a few years away. Others have shown dramatic success in animal studies, but require more work before advancing to clinical trials.

Antiangiogenesis

In order for tumors to grow, they must recruit new blood vessels—a process called angiogenesis—to meet increased energy demands. If these new blood vessels can be prevented, the tumor's size will stabilize or decrease, giving other treatments an opportunity to kill the cancerous cells.

Research on antiangiogenic drugs began in the 1970s, but it was not until the mid-1990s that clinical trials tested this approach as a cancer treatment. The trials involved thalidomide, the notorious morning sickness drug developed in Europe in the 1950s that resulted in a large number of birth defects, mainly characterized by malformed arms and legs. Dr. Judah Folkman, a professor at Harvard Medical School, recognized that thalidomide had caused these defects by retarding the growth of new blood vessels critical to embryonic limb buds. He hypothesized that thalidomide would have the same effect on cancer cells, slowing the growth of blood vessels that are necessary for cancer cells to survive and multiply.

The clinical trials tested thalidomide's effect on prostate cancer, Kaposi's sarcoma, glioblastoma, and multiple myeloma. EntreMed, a small biotechnology company, funded Dr. Folkman's research in exchange for the rights to the drugs he developed or discovered. While trial results fell short of establishing thalidomide as a highly effective treatment for cancer, they showed that it has some efficacy. For example, the glioblastoma trial found that 50 percent of patients with recurrent disease had their tumors stabilize or regress for significant periods of time.[2] A later trial that combined thalidomide with carboplatin reported regression or stabilization rates of 60 to 70 percent.[3] Given that the median survival time for patients with recurrent glioblastoma is three to four months, thalidomide represents an improvement; however, the great majority of patients treated with thalidomide eventually have a recurrence and die from their disease.

Currently, thalidomide is the only available prescription drug with published clinical data supporting its use as an antiangiogenic agent. It received FDA approval as a treatment for leprosy because of a second effect: the suppression of an inflammatory cytokine called tumor necrosis factor. This property makes thalidomide an effective treatment for a variety of autoimmune diseases, including Crohn's disease and lupus. Because drugs approved for any purpose can be prescribed for other diseases at a physician's discretion, thalidomide is now widely used by cancer patients, even though phase-III cancer trials have never been conducted.

The mechanism by which thalidomide suppresses the growth of new blood vessels is presently unknown; however, there is a great deal of information about the process of angiogenesis, and this knowledge provides the basis for the many new drugs on the horizon. At last count, at least twenty such drugs are under development, and some of these have advanced to phase-II clinical trials.

In developing antiangiogenic agents, most drug companies have tried to identify protein "growth factors," which are emitted by cancer cells. The growth factors direct blood vessel cells to initiate new growth in the direction of the tumor cells. Blood vessel cells, like all cells, have specific protein receptors on their surface. These receptors allow growth factors to enter the blood vessel cells and create internal changes that cause the cells to replicate. One way to prevent the growth of new blood vessels is to disable this signaling system, either by neutralizing the growth factors secreted by cancer cells or blocking the receptors on the surface of blood vessel cells.

There are multiple growth factors involved in the creation of new blood vessels, including fibroblast growth factor, platelet-derived growth factor, and vascular endothelial growth factor (VEGF). VEGF appears to be the most important, and drugs that target it seem to be more successful than those that target other growth factors. However, any drug that targets only one, or perhaps even two or three, growth factors may have only partial success. Cancer cells mutate and evolve, emitting whatever growth factors are needed for survival. Thus, even if a drug completely inhibits the VEGF signaling system, cancer cells may increase the secretion of other growth factors to compensate for the loss.

Judah Folkman and his collaborators decided to attack angiogenesis from a different angle.[4] They observed that surgical removal of the primary tumor is often followed by the rapid growth of metastatic tumors elsewhere in the body. This suggests that the primary tumor somehow suppresses the growth of satellite metastases. Folkman hypothesized that the primary tumor, or the body in response to the primary tumor, secretes one or more agents that inhibit metastatic tumor growth. He eventually determined that these inhibitory agents were Angiostatin and Endostatin, complex proteins initially isolated from the urine of mice but now produced through recombinant DNA techniques. When these drugs were injected into laboratory mice with implanted tumors, the results were the most astounding ever reported in cancer research.[5] Endostatin alone regressed several different types of tumors. Regression continued until administration was suspended, which allowed the tumors to regrow. When administration was resumed, tumor regression occurred again. This pattern of growth and regression was repeated for up to seven cycles. Finally, administration of Endostatin was continued until the tumor was no longer evident. When the drug was then discontinued, tumor growth did not recur. Other studies showed that a combination of Angiostatin and Endostatin not only created a marked increase in tumor regression, but required much smaller dosages than Endostatin alone.[6] Moreover, no toxicity was evident with either drug. Subsequent studies using very high dosages of Endostatin in monkeys have confirmed the absence of detectable toxicity.

The ability to modulate tumor growth through cycles of drug therapy without creating toxicity or diminishing the effectiveness of the drug heralds a new age in cancer treatment. It may overcome one of the critical problems in treatment today: drug resistance. Many chemotherapy agents are somewhat effective at first, but they quickly lose their effectiveness with repeated administration. Like HIV, cancerous cells attempt to ensure their survival by mutating quickly and

SURVIVING "TERMINAL" CANCER

adapting to their environment. This high mutation rate combined with a high rate of cell division makes it difficult for any single drug to retain its effectiveness. But Angiostatin and Endostatin do not target cancer cells. They target endothelial cells, of which new blood vessels are composed. Endothelial cells mutate slowly, if at all, so they do not develop resistance to the drugs. Thus, Angiostatin and Endostatin can stop endothelial cells from replicating, preventing the growth of new blood vessels. This starves the cancer cells regardless of their attempts to adjust to new environmental demands. Like Napoleon's army in Russia, the ferocity of the cancer cell is irrelevant if there is no energy to sustain its advances.

It remains to be seen whether Angiostatin and Endostatin will be as effective clinically as they have been in laboratory experiments. Both are currently under study in human clinical trials. Phase-I results for Endostatin were reported in November 2000: three of sixty patients who received the drug had significant tumor regression, and another dozen or so had stabilization. At first glance, this result seems less than spectacular, but recall that phase-I trials use dose escalation, so many of the patients began with insufficient dosages. Moreover, the method of administration (daily intravenous infusions) was different from the method used in animal experiments (subcutaneous injections). With the latter method, the drug is absorbed into the blood stream at a much slower rate, and it remains in the body for longer periods of time. New clinical trials are now underway using both subcutaneous injections and continuous low-dosage infusion pumps. Folkman had advocated these methods from the beginning but was overruled by the FDA and National Cancer Institute.

Despite the drugs' lack of toxicity, and despite evidence that they are at least ten times more effective when combined, bureaucratic rules require Angiostatin and Endostatin to be studied separately before they can be tested in combination. Those who make such rules clearly share none of the sense of urgency endured by cancer patients desperately in need of an effective treatment. If our roles were reversed, I doubt that any of them would hesitate to enroll in a trial that combined the two drugs, regardless of whether preliminary investigations had been made.

Because of clinical trial protocols required by the FDA, it will take another one to two years before these drugs become available. In the meantime, oncologists who advocate antiangiogenesis treatment are beginning to develop antiangiogenic cocktails using available drugs that were developed for other purposes. Celebrex and Vioxx, cox-2 inhibitors used to treat arthritis, and rosiglitazone (Avandia), developed for type-II diabetes, are now known to have significant antiangiogenic properties. Some oncologists are combining these drugs with thalidomide and chemotherapy. Because such efforts are very new, clinical outcome data has not yet been reported.

A variety of other treatment agents, many of which do not require a prescription, are also known to have antiangiogenic effects. These include tamoxifen,[7] gamma-linolenic acid,[8] genistein,[9] green tea,[10] curcumin,[11] vitamin D_3,[12] and silymarin (a supplement derived from milk thistle, commonly used for liver detoxification).[13] Not coincidentally, I had identified several of these agents early on as potential components of my multifaceted treatment program.

Different agents may have different mechanisms for preventing angiogenesis. As yet, these mechanisms are largely unknown. It seems feasible, however, that combining agents will create a synergistic effect. For example, one study showed that the combination of thalidomide and sulindac (an anti-inflammatory drug used for arthritis) produced a greater antiangiogenic effect than either agent alone.[14] In addition, laboratory research has shown that even small dosages of antiangiogenic drugs can greatly increase the effectiveness of both radiation and chemotherapy.[15,16] By preventing the recruitment of blood vessels, these drugs are believed to block cellular repair mechanisms that cancer cells need to overcome the cytotoxic effects of traditional treatments. Such combinations could have major clinical benefits, but, as

SURVIVING "TERMINAL" CANCER

discussed in previous chapters, combinational treatments are low on the agenda of conventional cancer research, so cancer patients need to develop their own combinations. Fortunately, most of the agents discussed in this chapter can be obtained by any cancer patient, albeit with some difficulty.

Antiangiogenic agents could potentially be combined with copper-depleting agents. Recent studies have shown that copper is required for the construction of new blood vessels. Agents (and diets) that produce low levels of copper in the body may therefore retard angiogenesis. Dr. George Brewer and collaborators at the University of Michigan have developed a copper-depleting chemical compound called ammonium tetrathiomolybdate (TM) for the treatment of Wilson's disease, a genetic, sometimes fatal disorder that causes dangerously high concentrations of copper in various organs of the body. (TM is manufactured by the Aldrich Chemical Company and is much cheaper than most prescription drugs.) Dr. Brewer has also used zinc acetate as a copper-depleting agent. Both drugs are relatively nontoxic.[17] In an ongoing clinical trial, eighteen patients with advanced metastatic cancer (and a life expectancy of less than three months) received enough TM to maintain their copper levels within a range that did not produce clinical side effects.[18] Six of the eighteen patients achieved stabilization. Subsequent studies using a higher dosage of TM have resulted in even higher response rates.

Inhibition of Cell Signaling Channels

All cells contain growth factor receptors, which allow them to receive signals that tell them to divide. But cancerous cells often develop mutations that cause these receptors to multiply wildly, producing a high rate of cell division.

One category of growth factors is a class of proteins known as tyrosine kinases, which includes the epidermal growth factor (EPGF). A significant percentage of cancers have an overabundance of EPGF receptors, including about half of glioblastomas and almost all squamous cell cancers.

Two strategies have been used to combat the explosive malignant growth caused by an overabundance of EPGF receptors. The first is to construct monoclonal antibodies either to combine with these receptors, preventing the growth factor from entering the cell body, or to attach to the cell, killing it with a toxin or a small radiation load (radioactive iodine much like that used in the treatment of thyroid cancer). Several versions of this treatment have been studied. At Hahnemann University in Philadelphia, researchers intravenously administered monoclonal antibodies targeting the EPGF receptors in glioblastoma patients.[19] Because the monoclonal antibodies were loaded with radioactive iodine, they were expected to kill any cancerous cells with which they had contact. Results of this study, however, were not easily interpretable. Though a small number of patients had significant tumor regression, median survival times were unimpressive. This may have been due to the fact that only half of glioblastoma tumors have an overabundance of EPGF receptors. Also, monoclonal antibodies are large molecules, and it is difficult for them to cross the blood-brain barrier in order to contact all of the malignant cells.

Monoclonal antibody treatment has been more successful with squamous cell skin cancers. In one trial, antibodies designed to block the EPGF receptors were used with standard chemotherapy. The combination completely eliminated malignancy for over 90 percent of trial participants,[20] and sponsors of the trial noted that monoclonal antibody treatment could help a wide spectrum of cancer patients.

A second approach in combating the malignant effects of tyrosine kinase activity is to use small molecules that mimic the epidermal growth factor without stimulating the EPGF receptors to respond to the signal. While pharmaceutical companies are developing synthetic versions, such molecules are already present in 13-*cis*-retinoic acid (otherwise known as Accutane or isotretinoin) and genistein (an isoflavone found in soy), both of which are potent inhibitors of tyrosine kinase activity.

Another growth factor that stimulates the replication of some cancerous cells is protein kinase C. Tamoxifen is a known protein kinase C inhibitor, but many other inhibitors are under development, and some of these are likely to be even more effective. Combining agents that target either protein kinase C or the epidermal growth factor might produce synergistic inhibitory effects.

In addition to growth factor receptors, cancer cells have an overabundance of interleukin receptors. Interleukins are cytokines that increase the immune system's inflammatory reaction to foreign proteins. By attaching a cytotoxic agent to particular interleukins, it should be possible to target and kill specific cancer cells. This strategy is under investigation in clinical trials with glioblastoma patients. Glioblastomas have interleukin-4 and interleukin-13 receptors, which are much more prevalent on cancer cells than on normal brain cells. In one clinical trial, a toxin from *Pseudomonas* (a common bacteria that causes pneumonia, bladder infections, and other infections) was fused with interleukin-4, then injected into the tumor area via an intracranial catheter. This produced significant tumor necrosis in five of the first seven patients who received the treatment;[21] however, the degree of necrosis caused life-threatening edema. Laboratory research suggests that interleukin-13 receptors are much more specific to glioma cells than interleukin-4 receptors, and therefore should be safer. Clinical trials targeting interleukin-13 receptors are now in progress.

STI-571, now known as Gleevec, is by far the most successful example of growth factor inhibition. Developed for a relatively rare form of leukemia, it targets a particular receptor on the leukemia cells and has had almost 90 to 100 percent success in arresting malignancy.[22]

Monoclonal Antibodies

Targeting growth factor receptors is one of many uses for monoclonal antibodies. Whenever cancer cells have proteins that differentiate them from normal cells, monoclonal antibodies can be constructed to target those proteins, thus selectively killing the cancer cells with either radiation or a toxin. This approach, however, often yields disappointing results. First, it requires that the proteins targeted by monoclonal antibodies be highly specific to the cancer cell. Otherwise, normal cells will also be damaged. Second, to kill a tumor, the monoclonal antibodies must make contact with all the cancer cells. This may or may not occur depending on the site of the tumor and the tumor's blood supply.

In an earlier chapter, I described my interest in monoclonal antibodies as a treatment for my brain tumor. Developed in Italy,[23] this treatment was being tested by Dr. Henry Friedman at Duke University. Dr. Friedman used monoclonal antibodies to target an extracellular protein known as tenascin. The function of tenascin is largely unknown, although it is found on some normal adult cells and is present during embryonic and fetal development. High levels of tenascin are found on the cells of many kinds of cancer; and higher levels seem to indicate a worse prognosis. Among brain tumors, for example, glioblastomas have much more tenascin than lower-grade gliomas. A similar correlation has been reported for different grades of cervical cancer. To be considered for Dr. Friedman's treatment, I was required to send in histology blocks of my tumor so he could evaluate my tenascin levels. My tumor passed this test with flying colors, confirming my poor prognosis.

I eventually declined to participate in Duke's clinical trial because I became convinced that the configuration of my tumor made me a poor candidate for the treatment. My tumor was very large, and it was spread out over two separate areas. It seemed unlikely that the antibodies would make contact with all the tumor cells. Moreover, glioma cells extend beyond the observable boundaries of the tumor bed. While the radiation could kill cells adjacent to those contacted by the mono-clonal antibodies, cells that were just a short distance away would be unaffected. Like all localized approaches to brain tumor treatment, this procedure might have retarded my tumor growth, but I believed it was unlikely to have a long-term benefit.

A somewhat different use of monoclonal antibodies is to target the dead tissue that typically develops at the center of a glioblastoma. The tumor's rapid growth outward draws energy away from cells in the center, causing these cells to die. Monoclonal antibodies loaded with radioactive iodine can target this dead tissue, providing a dose of radiation to the living cancer cells that surround it. This procedure should be more effective the more often it is given, because each treatment kills the living cells adjacent to the dead tissue, creating an even larger target for the next round of treatment.[24]

The general inaccessibility of brain tumors poses a problem for monoclonal antibody treatment. Other cancers may be treated more successfully; however, researchers must surmount one very important problem: tumor cells in different individuals have their own specific antigens, which makes it difficult to construct a monoclonal antibody that works for everyone. One tactic is to develop monoclonal antibodies for individual patients, but this is expensive and time consuming. Moreover, it does not guarantee success, because individuals may have different antigen patterns on the different components of their tumor. Another tactic is to construct monoclonal antibodies that target an average antigen pattern within a diagnostic category. This means that the treatment will be more effective for some people than for others. There are now over one hundred generic monoclonal antibodies corresponding to different antigen sets. Two of these, one for B-cell lymphoma and one for breast cancer, have received FDA approval for cancer treatment. Six others have been approved for noncancer purposes.

Herceptin, approved for breast cancer, illustrates both the promise and limitations of monoclonal antibody treatment. Among breast cancer patients, 25 to 30 percent have an overabundance of HER2 oncogene receptors. HER2 oncogene is a tyrosine kinase related to the epidermal growth factor discussed on page 241 and 242. When Herceptin combines with the HER2 oncogene receptors, it inhibits cancer cell growth by reducing the signals for cell division. It also increases sensitivity to chemotherapy by inhibiting cellular repair mechanisms.

Patients who can benefit from Herceptin are identified by immunoassay. Tailoring treatments according to individual characteristics will be an important tool in the future, but in this instance, results have been less than dramatic. In one phase-II trial, Herceptin was given to metastatic breast cancer patients who failed standard treatment; 10 to 15 percent of the patients had tumor regression and 30 percent had stabilization.[25] Another study, which combined Herceptin with chemotherapy, increased the percentage of patients with tumor regression and approximately doubled the stabilization period, but many patients still received no benefit from the treatment.[26] The mixed outcome presumably reflected the variability of protein antigens among patients.

Similar results have occurred with monoclonal antibodies that target B-cell lymphoma. Approximately 50 percent of patients have tumor regression with an extended survival time.[27] Like Herceptin, this treatment constitutes a meaningful improvement, but it obviously is not a magic bullet.

Gene Therapy

Cancer is a disease of the genes, occurring because of aberrations in the DNA code. Whereas normal genes cause cells to grow until they differentiate into specialized functions, the oncogenes of cancer cells produce cell division at a rapid rate, and the cells remain in a somewhat primitive, undifferentiated state, not unlike fetal cells.

In principle, cancer could be effectively treated by identifying the nature of the genetic defect, then inserting normal genes to replace the defective ones. This approach has been investigated for more than a decade, but results have been disappointing. Such treatments require an enormous amount of information about the underlying genetic defects, a means of manufacturing genes that exactly mimic the naturally occurring genes (otherwise cancer cells may simply disregard them), and the technology to insert the replacement genes in all the tumor cells. Progress is being made, however, and much more is expected now that the Human Genome Project has provided the complete genetic sequencing of all our chromosomes. In the next five to ten years, we will have a detailed understanding of the genetic basis for many kinds of cancer. Unfortunately, the FDA's approval process will delay access to gene therapy treatments, and many people who have cancer today will not live to see these developments reach fruition.

In brain cancer trials, researchers have inserted genes with known properties into cancer cells, endowing the cancer cells with specific features that make them targets for therapeutic agents. For example, one set of trials used a modified herpes virus that was engineered to infect actively dividing cells. Since normal cells do not routinely divide, only the cancer cells were infected with the virus. The infected cells were then killed with antiviral drugs.

There were two limitations to this treatment. First, the herpes virus was engineered so it could not replicate on its own (to prevent encephalitis). This meant that the amount of virus available was limited to that which was directly injected. Second, since the virus only infected cells that were in the process of division, cancerous cells that were not dividing were not infected. Despite these limitations, several laboratory experiments produced major, sometimes complete, tumor regression after using this treatment in rodents. When cells were killed by gene therapy, they exerted a "bystander effect," killing a large percentage of surrounding cells not infected by the virus. Also, many uninfected cells died even when they were not adjacent to the infected cells. This indicates that the immune system created antibodies to the antigens of infected cancer cells, and these antibodies generalized to the uninfected cells because of their genetic similarity.

When I began my search for treatment, phase-I trials for gene therapy had just begun. I called two of the universities conducting these trials to inquire about the problems and benefits they had observed. I was told that several patients had significant tumor regression persisting for several months; however, few, if any, had been cured, and most patients received minimal benefits.

The clinical trial results were published in 1998, three years after my initial inquiry, and they confirmed the information I had been given.[28] Of twelve patients with recurrent glioblastoma, the median survival time was 206 days, and 25 percent of the patients survived longer than twelve months. Four months after treatment, four patients had no recurrence. Their median survival time was 528 days, compared with 194 days for patients who did have a recurrence. Of the former group, one patient still had not had a recurrence nearly three years after treatment. Clearly, gene therapy is no panacea, but remember that the median survival time for glioblastoma patients who are treated after recurrence is three to five months; of these, very few patients enjoy long-term survival. Thus, gene therapy does show promise, and refinements of the procedure might produce even more positive results. Unfortunately, the sponsor of the clinical trial, Novartis Pharmaceuticals, has abandoned the project because it did not think the results were promising enough to be profitable.

A new approach to cancer treatment, based on recombinant DNA technology, is called antisense gene therapy. In this treatment, an artificially constructed gene containing antisense DNA (which neutralizes any targeted segment of DNA) is inserted into cancer cells. While details of the treatment are beyond the scope of this book, there is no doubt that antisense technology can prevent the aberrant genes of cancer cells from causing malignant growth. For example, researchers at M.D. Anderson Cancer Center used antisense technology to target the vascular endothelial growth factor (VEGF) necessary for angiogenesis (see page 237). They used a recombinant adenovirus, the same virus that causes the common cold, to carry the antisense DNA into cancer cells. The DNA was expected to disable the gene that caused VEGF production. When tested on mice with actively growing glioblastomas, this gene insertion method substantially inhibited tumor growth.[29]

Immunological Treatments

Because cancer cells have a genetic structure different from normal cells, they generate foreign proteins. These proteins should be detected by the immune system, evoking the same reaction as any foreign virus or bacteria. Yet, the immune system fails to do its job. There are two known reasons for this.

First, cancer cells secrete enzymes and proteins that suppress the immunological detection system. This is especially true for glioblastomas, which use at least three different cloaking mechanisms. In order to be effective, immunological cancer treatments must surmount these tumor defense mechanisms. To date, however, relatively little progress has been made, although a variety of new approaches are being studied.

Second, a weakened immune system may not be effective in fighting cancer cells. For example, AIDS patients contract many different diseases, including cancer, because their immune systems have been severely weakened by the HIV virus. Similarly, older cancer patients often have a worse prognosis than younger cancer patients, who tend to have stronger immune systems. All of this suggests that cancer might be successfully treated simply by boosting the patient's immune system. This is the rationale behind broad-spectrum boosters such as interferons. (Interferon treatment, in fact, has been somewhat effective, especially for melanoma. It also has shown an effect on brain tumors, although benefits are usually short-lived.) Melatonin, various mushroom extracts, and Poly-ICLC also seem to strengthen the immune system. Such agents may be worthwhile adjuncts to any cancer treatment, especially if they are nontoxic.

Immunological treatments have an immediate appeal, because many cancer patients believe they will be easier to tolerate than chemotherapy. Rather than poison the body, would it not be better to strengthen its defenses against disease? This is one of the major principles of alternative medicine, which decries the debilitating effects of standard cancer treatments.

Unfortunately, immunological treatments are not necessarily benign. Interferon treatment, for example, creates an inflammatory effect not unlike a bad allergic reaction. When inflammation is too severe, it can be fatal. The same problem occurs with other agents that increase immunoreactivity, especially the inflammatory cytokines. These include tumor necrosis factor and the various interleukins. Interleukin-2 is perhaps the most common—and among the most potent.

In 1995, *Cancer* published a study on an immunological treatment for recurrent brain tumors, mainly glioblastomas.[30] The white blood cells of a brain tumor patient were mixed with the white blood cells of an unrelated donor, then incubated for several days. This created "angry white blood cells," lymphocyte killer cells that generated an array of inflammatory cytokines. These cells were combined with interleukin-2, then infused into the patient's tumor bed through an intracranial catheter. Patients received this regimen regularly until disease progression became evident. The treatment produced a median survival time of fifty-three weeks. (When recurrent tumors are treated with chemotherapy, the expected survival time is three to four months.) The authors noted that results might have been more positive if patients had received the treatment immediately after diagnosis. At the time of recurrence, most patients had already received chemotherapy, which presumably had weakened their immune systems. The authors argued that immunotherapy should be the first treatment option and chemotherapy should be reserved until immunotherapy fails.

A somewhat different immunological approach uses a technique that amplifies the T cell levels in cancer patients. In one study, glioblastoma cells gathered during surgery were cultured in the presence of growth factors, then injected subcutaneously back into the patient. After an immunological reaction developed, lymphocytes attacking the tumor cells were removed from the patient's lymph nodes. These were then cultured with a staphylococcus toxin and a low dose of interleukin-2. This generated a large number of activated T cells, which were then presented to the patient by intravenous infusion. Of the ten patients participating in the trial, two enjoyed tumor regression, with regression persisting in one patient at the time the study was published (over seventeen months after the treatment). Of the eight patients with progressive disease, four were alive after one year, suggesting that the treatment had some benefits aside from tumor regression.[31]

The holy grail of immunotherapy is the development of effective cancer vaccines. This should be possible because of differences between the protein structures of cancer cells and normal cells. While some progress has been made, especially with respect to melanoma, cancer vaccines have been disappointing in general. As with monoclonal antibodies, the fundamental problem is that different people have different antigens, so generic vaccines will not work for everyone. For this reason, the development of patient-specific vaccines is now the primary focus of immunotherapy research.

Another area of active investigation is the effort to increase the detectability of tumor antigens. As noted earlier, tumors secrete enzymes that essentially provide a protective cloak for these antigens. The larger the tumor, the stronger its defense against immune-system detection. (For this reason, cancer vaccines seem to work best when tumors are small.) The most promising method for overcoming this defense mechanism is the use of dendritic cells. Derived from bone marrow, dendritic cells have been characterized as "professional antigen-presented cells." They are cultured with cells taken from the patient's tumor, and this culture is stimulated with granulocyte-macrophage colony-stimulating factor (GM-CSF) and interleukin-4. (GM-CSF is the growth factor used to counteract the decrease in white-blood-cell counts caused by chemotherapy.) When the mixture is injected into the patient, it evokes an increased reaction from the immune system. This procedure has substantially increased the survival time for rats with gliomas.[32] It is now under investigation in human clinical trials.

———

Some of these new treatment modalities, such as monoclonal antibodies and cancer vaccines, are showing incremental progress, while others, such as the antiangiogenic drugs, have produced dramatic success in laboratory experiments, though this success has not yet been replicated in clinical trials. The fact that these treatments are well along in the clinical trial process is cause for optimism. With any luck, some of them will bring major improvements in the way cancer is treated in the near future.

ENDNOTES

1. Smith, T. J., et al. Efficacy and cost effectiveness of cancer treatment: rational allocation of resources based on decision analysis. *Journal of the National Cancer Institute.* 1993;85(18):1460-1474.

2. Fine, H., et al. A phase-II trial of the anti-angiogenic agent, thalidomide, in patients with recurrent high-grade gliomas. *Proceedings of the American Society for Clinical Oncology.* 1997;abstract 1372.

3. Glass, J., et al. Phase-I/II study of carboplatin and thalidomide in recurrent glioblastoma multiforme. *Proceedings of the American Society for Clinical Oncology.* 1999;abstract 551.

4. The story of Folkman's twenty-year struggle to develop antiangiogenic treatments for cancer is chronicled in a *Dr. Folkman's War* (New York: Random House; 2000) by noted science writer Robert Cooke.

5. Boehm, T., et al. Antiangiogenic therapy of experimental cancer does not induce acquired drug resistance. *Nature*. 1997;390(6658):404-407.

6. Yokoyama, Y., et al. Synergy between Angiostatin and Endostatin: inhibition of ovarian cancer. *Cancer Research*. 2000;60(8):2190-2196.

7. Gagliardi, A. R., et al. Antiestrogens inhibit endothelial cell growth stimulated by angiogenic growth factors. *Anticancer Research*. 1996;16(3A):1101-1106.

8. Cai, J., et al. Inhibition of angiogenic factor- and tumour-induced angiogenesis by gamma linolenic acid. *Prostaglandins, Leukotrienes and Essential Fatty Acids*. 1999;60(1):21-29.

9. Zhou, J. R., et al. Soybean phytochemicals inhibit the growth of transplantable human prostate carcinoma and tumor angiogenesis in mice. *Journal of Nutrition*. 1999;129(9):1628-1635.

10. Cao, Y., and Cao, R. Angiogenesis inhibited by drinking tea. *Nature*. 1998;392:381.

11. Arbiser, J. L., et al. Curcumin is an in vivo inhibitor of angiogenesis. *Molecular Medicine*. 1998;4(6):376-383.

12. Majewski, S., et al. Vitamin D_3 is a potent inhibitor of tumor cell-induced angiogenesis. Symposium Proceedings. *Journal of Investigative Dermatology*. 1996;1(1):97-101.

13. Jiang, C., et al. Anti-angiogenic potential of a cancer chemopreventive flavonoid antioxidant, silymarin: inhibition of key attributes of vascular endothelial cells and angiogenic cytokine secretions by cancer epithelial cells. *Biochemical and Biophysical Research Communications*. 2000;276(1):371-378.

14. Verheul, H. M., et al. Combination oral antiangiogenic therapy with thalidomide and sulindac inhibits tumor growth in rabbits. *British Journal of Cancer*. 1999;79(1):114-118.

15. In animal studies, low doses of Angiostatin given immediately after radiation treatment greatly increased the cytotoxic effect of the radiation. (Gorski, D. H., et al. Potentiation of the antitumor effect of ionizing radiation by brief concomitant exposures to Angiostatin. *Cancer Research*. 1998;58[24]:5686-5689.)

16. When squalamine (a new antiangiogenic agent derived from the liver of dogfish) was combined with cisplatin, the cytotoxic effect on ovarian cancer

cells substantially increased. (Pietras, R. J., et al. Squalamine and cisplatin block angiogenesis and growth of ovarian cancer cells with and without overexpression of HER-2/neu oncogene. *Proceedings of the American Association for Cancer Research.* 1999;abstract 398.)

17. If copper levels become too low, existing blood vessels may be damaged. Patients using copper-depleting agents should have their hematocrit and white-blood-cell count monitored as well as their level of ceruloplasmin, a glycoprotein that transports serum copper.

18. Fox, Maggie. Copper-lowering drug may fight cancer. Reuters News Service. 2000 Jan 20.

19. Snelling, L., et al. Epidermal growth factor receptor 425 monoclonal antibodies radiolabeled with iodine-125 in the adjuvant treatment of high-grade astrocytomas. *Hybridroma.* 1995;14(2):111-114.

20. ImClone Systems Incorporated press release, 1999 May 17.

21. Neurocrine Biosciences press release, 1998 Nov 25.

22. Leukemia drug heralds molecularly targeted era. *Journal of the National Cancer Institute.* 2000;92(1):6-8.

23. Riva, P., et al. 131I radioconjugated antibodies for the locoregional radioimmunotherapy of high-grade malignant glioma: phase-I and -II study. *Acta Oncologica.* 1999;38(3):351-359.

24. Techniclone Corporation press release, 1997 May 19.

25. Baselga, J., et al. Phase-II study of weekly intravenous trastuzumab (Herceptin) in patients with HER2/neu-overexpressing metastatic breast cancer. *Seminars in Oncology.* 1999;26(4 suppl 12):78-83.

26. Pegram, M. D., et al. Phase-II study of receptor-enhanced chemosensitivity using recombinant humanized anti-p185HER2/neu monoclonal antibody plus cisplatin in patients with HER2/neu-overexpressing metastatic breast cancer refractory to chemotherapy treatment. *Journal of Clinical Oncology.* 1998;16(8):2659-2671.

27. Grillo-Lopez, A. J., et al. Overview of the clinical development of rituximab: first monoclonal antibody approved for the treatment of lymphoma. *Seminars in Oncology.* 1999;26(5 suppl 4):66-73.

28. Klatzmann, D., et al. A phase-I/II study of herpes simplex virus type I thymidine kinase "suicide" gene therapy for recurrent glioblastoma. Study Group on Gene Therapy for Glioblastoma. *Human Gene Therapy.* 1998;9(17):2595-2604.

29. Im, S. A., et al. Antiangiogenesis treatment for gliomas: transfer of antisense-vascular endothelial growth factor inhibits tumor growth in vivo. *Cancer Research.* 1999;59(4):895-900.

30. Hayes, R. L., et al. Improved long-term survival after intracavitary interleukin-2 and lymphokine-activated killer cells for adults with recurrent malignant glioma. *Cancer.* 1995;76(5):840-852.

31. Plautz, E. G., et al. Systemic T cell adoptive immunotherapy of malignant gliomas. *Journal of Neurosurgery.* 1998;89(1):42-51.

32. Liau, L. M., et al. Treatment of intracranial gliomas with bone marrow-derived dendritic cells used with tumor antigens. *Journal of Neurosurgery.* 1999;90(6):1115-1124.

Sources of Information

CANCER PATIENTS WOULD BE FOOLISH TO RELY ENTIRELY ON THE recommendations of their oncologists. As discussed in earlier chapters, a number of circumstances govern the advice that oncologists provide, and some of these conflict with the patients' best interests. It is therefore essential that patients or their loved ones do their own research and locate additional treatment options. This chapter offers a brief description of different sources of information on the Internet. The list is by no means exhaustive, as the Internet can provide detailed information on every conceivable topic. The problem is determining which information is credible and useful and finding sources you can trust.

The advantage to using the World Wide Web is that many Web sites provide links to other sites. Thus, once a useful site is found, it can lead to enormous amounts of information. For help with Internet research, try www.whatsonthe.net. You might also consider Susan Detwiler's book, *Super Searchers on Health and Medicine: The Online Secrets of Top Health and Medical Researchers* (Medford, N.J.: Cyberage, 2000).

The first stop for any cancer patient should be www.cancerguide.org. Steve Dunn, the organizer, is a cancer survivor with great insight into the needs of cancer patients and offers methods to facilitate patients' research. A thorough exploration of his Web site and its links will go a long way toward providing cancer patients with basic but essential information.

For brain cancer patients, Al Musella's www.virtualtrials.com is an abundant resource, providing information about new treatments and clinical trials. It, too, has numerous links, including a listserv called the BrainTmr group, which I referenced earlier.

For information about complementary and alternative medicine, try www.rosenthal.hs.columbia.edu/Guide6.html, which is maintained by the Rosenthal Center. For information about nutritional supplements and general health news, visit The Life Extension Foundation at www.lef.org.

Information found on the Internet is rarely firsthand. It is often inaccurate, and it is not necessarily current with breaking developments. To obtain the most accurate information, go to PubMed, a free service available at www.pubmedcentral.nih.gov. PubMed posts abstracts of current articles published in the primary medical journals. The journal articles are usually based on research that was completed one to two years earlier. At this time in history, when new treatments are being introduced at an unprecedented rate, this lag time can mean life or death for cancer patients in the terminal stages of their disease. For the most current information about new treatments, refer to reports from the major cancer conferences, including annual meetings of the American Association for Cancer Research and the American Society of Clinical Oncology. Abstracts of the papers presented at annual meetings are available at the organizations' respective Web sites: www.aacr.org and www.asco.org. These abstracts often provide information about new treatments as well as the locations of clinical trials. Whenever possible, contact the oncologists conducting these trials to learn the details about the treatments and any results that may be available.

Finally, Medscape provides monthly updates on the cutting edge of new medical treatments, including breaking developments from journal articles and professional meetings. For a free subscription, go to http://oncology.medscape.com.

Index

abstracts, medical, 31, 33, 90, 94, 115, 123, 132-133, 200, 252, 254, 258

Accutane, 51-52, 55, 87, 89, 93, 101-102, 115-117, 120, 129, 162, 165, 243; side effects of, 51, 120; mechanism of action, 88

ACNU, 48, 216, 230.

activism, patient, 163, 169

Adderbrooke Hospital, 220

adenovirus, 249

adhesion molecules, 219

age, 2, 43, 103, 118-119, 122, 146-147, 149-150, 152-153, 155-158, 174, 197, 212, 238

Agent Orange, 9

aging, 207, 212

AIDS, 86-87, 117, 163, 216, 249

AIDS cocktail, 88, 163

alcohol, 7, 11, 50, 55, 202, 219, 225, 235

Aldrich Chemical Company, 241

Allen, Woody, 43

allergic reaction, 250

alpha-linoleic acid, 217

alpha tocopherol, 209, 228

alternative medicine, 3, 30, 114, 126, 141, 154, 166, 169, 171-187, 189, 191, 193, 195-199, 201, 203, 205-206, 210, 212-213, 227, 234-235, 250, 258

Alternative Medicine Definitive Guide to Cancer, 172, 177-178, 180, 182-184, 197-198

American Association of Cancer Research, 133, 200

American Brain Tumor Association, 57, 113

American Society of Clinical Oncology, 89, 94, 116, 258

amino acids, 186-187

ammonium tetrathiomolybdate (TM), 241

amygdalin. *See* laetrile.

Analysis of Variance, 157-158

anaplastic astrocytoma (AA-3), 20, 26, 33, 45, 85-86, 132, 153-155, 195

anaplastic oligoastrocytoma, 132

androgen-suppressive drugs, 174, 185, 214

anemia, 68

anesthesiologist, 19

angelica root, 211

angiogenesis, 93, 203, 215, 219, 223, 231, 235, 237-238, 240-241, 249, 253-254

Angiostatin, 94, 238-239, 253; side effects of, 238

animal experiments, 12, 14, 18, 46, 57, 62, 72, 82-83, 93, 96-97, 102, 105, 137, 178-179, 181, 188, 199-200, 203-205, 207, 210-211, 216, 218, 221-222, 224-226, 228-229, 231, 235, 238-239, 247, 249, 252-253, 255

animal rights movement, 72, 82

anthroposophy, 172, 180-181

anti-emetic drugs, 49

anti-inflammatory agents, 218, 230, 240

antiangiogenic drugs, 78-79, 89-92, 94, 236-237, 240-241, 252-253

antibodies, 29, 33, 36-37, 41, 48, 53, 116, 139-140, 143, 223, 242, 244-248, 251-252, 254

anticancer agents, 174, 177-178, 187, 199-200, 202, 211, 214, 220-223, 225-227, 229-231, 253. *See also* specific treatments.

anticonvulsant agents, 31-32

antigen, 29, 185, 213, 245-247, 251, 255

antineoplaston treatment, 33, 186-189, 191-195, 200

Antioxidant Miracle, The, 207, 228

brussels sprouts, 211, 226
Burdick, Dr. Robert, 191-192
Burr, Congressman Richard, 190
Burzynski Breakthrough, The, 186, 200
Burzynski, Dr. Stanislaw, 32-33, 186-195, 200
Bush, George, 226
bystander effect, 247

C-225, 139-140
cabbage, 226
cachexia, 179, 220
calcium channel blockers, 46-47
calmodulin antagonist, 93
Cambridge University, 220
Cameron, Dr. Ewan, 206, 227-228
Canada, 100, 123, 177, 180, 199
Canadian Medical Association, 177, 180, 199
cancer cells, 86, 88-89, 93, 139, 179,184, 187-188, 202-203, 210, 213, 216, 219, 223, 225-226, 236-237, 239-241, 244-249, 251, 253-254.
cancer community, 163, 186
cancer patient, 2-4, 49, 65-66, 70, 82, 89, 109-110, 118, 120, 126, 140, 142, 156, 161-165, 169, 173, 179, 183, 187, 191, 196, 198, 201, 204-206, 208, 211, 214-215, 220-221, 227-230, 234, 237, 239, 241-242, 246, 249-251, 257-258
cancer, 1, 3-4, 7-8, 20, 42, 51, 54-57, 62, 68, 75, 78-79, 82-83, 86-91, 93, 97, 99, 104-105, 110, 112-115, 117, 119-120, 122, 132-133, 135, 138-139, 141, 143, 145, 153, 157, 163-166, 169, 172, 174-188, 190-193, 196-210, 212-215, 217-231, 233-239, 241-255, 258; causes of, 8, 118, 205, 218, 233; prevention of; 115, 187, 201, 205-208, 217-218, 224, 226, 230-231; War on, 233-234. *See also* specific cancers.
Cantron, 184
carboplatin, 44, 48, 92, 94, 129, 133, 236, 252

carcinogen, 9, 173, 181, 216, 225, 228, 231-232
carmustine, 41
carrot juice, 36
case histories, 2, 31, 67, 98-99, 183, 191-192, 196-197
cataracts, 207
catheter, intracranial, 21, 38, 57, 243, 250
cauliflower, 226
CCNU, 41, 48, 55, 62
celandine, 182
Celebrex, 240
Celgene Corporation, 94
cell cultures, 57, 187-188, 210, 221
cell death, 200, 210-211, 228, 231, 245
cell differentiation, 88, 187, 210, 223, 244, 246
cell division, 46, 79, 88-89, 93, 139, 187, 223, 235, 239, 241, 246-247
cell membrane, 83, 93, 219, 221, 223
cellular matrix, 90
cerebral hemispheres, 13, 15, 37
ceruloplasmin levels, 254
cervical cancer, 183, 244
Chamberlain, Dr. Marc, 25-26, 31-37, 41-42, 45, 47-49, 51-53, 56, 58-59, 66, 68, 71, 73-74, 78-81, 89, 95-96, 116
cheese, 221
chelation, 173
chemotherapy, 25, 27, 34, 36-37, 40-41, 45-56, 58, 62, 64-69, 76, 87-89, 92, 101-104, 109, 113-115, 117, 119-120, 125, 127-129, 131-133, 139-140, 146, 151, 155-157, 164, 175-176, 182, 195, 197-200, 206, 209-210, 214-216, 219, 221, 226, 229, 231, 234, 238, 240, 242, 246, 250, 252, 254; controversy over, 174; potentiation of, 77, 88; side effects of, 49, 52, 55, 66, 175, 182. *See also* DNA damage.
Chen, Dr. Lichuan, 191
chi-square, 157
China, 225
Chinese herbs, 176
chiropractors, 172

Chlebowski, Dr. Rowan, 180, 196, 198
chlorinated water, 173
chlorpromazine, 62
cholesterol, 225
chronic myelogenous leukemia, 138
cis-platinum, 48
cisplatin, 199, 210, 214, 229, 253-254
citrus, 225
clinical trials. *See* trials.
cocktail, drug, 25, 35, 44, 48, 52, 54, 86-
    88, 92-93, 102-104, 110, 116-118,
    122, 129, 139, 161, 163, 165-166,
    172-173, 177, 183, 201, 210, 214,
    216, 220, 225, 230, 240-241, 243, 253
coenzyme Q10, 202, 208, 227
cognitive dysfunction, 64
cognitive test, 25
Coley's toxin, 184
colon cancer, 139, 198, 216, 218, 234
colorectal cancer, 175, 183, 198, 200,
    214, 216, 221, 224, 229-230, 235
complementary medicine, 166, 197. *See
    also* alternative medicine.
complete response to treatment, 54, 220
complex proteins, 203, 238
Congress, 82, 143, 176, 186, 190
conjugated linoleic acid (CLA), 221, 231
constipation, 68
contraindications, 88, 120
control group, 112-113, 119, 121-125,
    127, 140, 142, 145, 147-150, 154,
    157-158, 183, 196, 206, 211, 215-216
conventional medicine, 2-4, 92, 114, 118,
    124, 141, 162-163, 166, 171-177,
    182-186, 190-191, 195-197, 201,
    204-205, 210, 215, 217
coordination, 12
coping, 1, 3, 19, 50, 56, 68, 97-99, 213
copper, 241, 254
Coriolus versicolor, 215
corn oil, 217-218
corpus callosum, 37-38
cost of treatment, 30, 33, 42, 49, 51, 58,
    64, 72-73, 77, 82, 112-113, 139, 141-
    142, 147, 152, 154, 162-163, 190,
    203-205, 221, 227, 234, 252

cost-benefit ratio, 34, 45, 52, 57, 112,
    128, 131, 152, 164, 174-175, 203,
    221, 228, 248
Couldwell, Dr. William, 33-34, 42, 44,
    77, 132
cox inhibitors, 240
Cox Proportional Hazards Analysis, 157
cranberry juice, 21
Crime and Human Nature, 7
Crohn's disease, 141, 237
cruciferous, 211
curcumin, 227, 240, 253
cure, for cancer, 82, 85, 90, 92, 203,
    214, 233
cured, patients who are, 28, 69, 128, 178,
    197, 234, 248
cutting-edge treatments, 2-3, 104, 233,
    235, 237, 239, 241, 243, 245, 247,
    249, 251, 253, 255, 259
cyanide toxicity, 178
cytokines, 181, 213, 236, 243, 250, 253
cytotoxicity, 87, 156, 184, 200, 213, 215,
    221-222, 240, 243, 253

Dana-Farber Institute, 91
dandelion root, 211
dates, red, 211
DDT, 9
death, 1-3, 7-8, 13, 15, 20-21, 25, 31,
    34, 36, 42-43, 54, 56, 64-65, 67, 70,
    74, 76, 82, 86, 89, 96-97, 101-102,
    109, 118, 137-140, 161-162, 164-
    165, 179, 182, 191, 194, 219, 233-
    234, 236, 245, 258
debilitation, 3-4, 45, 97, 174, 178-179,
    250. *See also* cachexia.
defective gene, 156
dementia, 28
dendritic cells, 251, 255
Department of Agriculture, 234
depression, 3, 25, 31, 50, 55-56, 65, 96-
    97, 101, 110, 119, 177
detoxification, 173, 240
Detwiler, Susan, 257
DHEA, 227
diabetes, 221, 240

diagnosis, 1-3, 7, 11, 13-15, 17, 19, 21, 23, 25-27, 31, 44, 46-47, 56, 89, 97, 99-101, 103, 109, 132-133, 140, 142, 155, 161, 164-165, 172, 174, 191, 193-194, 199, 209, 234, 245, 250

diet, 20, 173-174, 176, 180, 182, 202, 204, 207, 209-211, 221, 223-226, 228-230, 235, 241

digestive system, 203

dihomo-gamma-linoleic acid, 217

Dilantin, 31

disoriented, 13

DNA, 207-208, 235, 238, 246, 248-249

docosahexaenoic acid (DHA), 217

dominance statistics, 158

dosage, 33, 41-42, 46, 49, 52, 58, 68, 76, 112, 115-116, 137, 173, 179, 181-182, 203, 206, 208, 210, 213-214, 221-222, 238-241

dose escalation, 137, 239

double-blind studies, 119, 199, 206

drug cocktail, 86, 88, 93, 102-104, 117, 163, 165

drug interactions, 88, 120

drug resistance, 2, 86-87, 104, 128, 156, 200, 226, 238-239, 253

drugs, storage of, 49, 51, 115

Duke University, 29, 193, 244

dura, 59, 61

early detection of cancer, 75, 234

edema, 21, 194, 243

EDTA, 173

effect size, 158

eicosapentenoic acid (EPA), 217, 219

elderly, 212, 219, 233

Elias, Thomas D., 186, 191, 200

emergency room, 14-15, 18, 21, 95

emotion, 1, 7, 21, 25, 31, 50, 53, 69, 74, 97, 180

Endostatin, 94, 137, 238-239, 253; side effects of, 137, 238

endothelial cells, 237, 239, 249, 253, 255

enemas, 173

England, 99-100, 125, 159, 220, 228

EntreMed, 91, 94, 236

epidemiological evidence, 202-203, 208-209, 221, 229-230

epidermal growth factor (EPGF), 241-243, 246; receptor, 88, 93, 139, 223, 231, 242, 254

epigallocatechin-3-gallate (EGCG), 225

epileptic seizures, 31

Erbitux (C-225), 139-140

error variance. *See* statistical noise.

esophageal cancer, 183

essiac tea, 176, 184

ethics, medical, 118, 135, 137, 139, 141, 143, 177

etoposide, 214, 229

Europe, 39, 78, 91, 105, 142, 176, 180, 202, 205, 213, 227, 236

evening primrose oil, 57, 220

exercise, 31, 207, 209, 235

experimental treatments, 113, 115, 118, 122-123, 127-129, 149-152, 154, 157-158

external beam radiation, 34

false negatives, 148

family history, 7, 205

fatigue, 48, 69

fatty acids, 57, 162, 165, 217-219, 221, 230-231, 253

federal law, 74

fetal blood vessels, 79, 91

fetal tissue, 75, 91, 244, 246

fiber bundle, 37

fibroblast growth factor, 237

Fine, Dr. Howard, 53, 91-92

first-line treatment, 104, 177, 214, 229

fish oil, 217-218, 220

5-fluorouracil, 183, 214, 229

flare imaging, 73, 75

flavonoids, 225, 253

flax seed oil, 217

Flor-Essence, 176, 184

fluorinated water, 173

folk medicine, 176. *See also* alternative medicine.

Folkman, Dr. Judah, 91, 93-94, 236, 238-239, 253

Food and Drug Administration (FDA), 4,
    33, 118, 123-124, 126-128, 131, 135-
    143, 145-146, 149, 153, 156-158,
    161-163, 166, 176, 188-191, 195,
    204-205, 239-240
Food and Drug Administration (FDA)
    approval, 4, 51, 112-114, 121, 123-
    127, 130, 132, 139, 141, 147, 188-
    189, 227, 236, 245, 247; criteria for,
    113, 121, 123-124, 126-127, 147,
    149, 158, 188
Food, Drug and Cosmetic Act, 142
foreign proteins, 213, 218, 243, 249
Framingham study, 202
free radicals, 88, 202, 207-210, 219
Freud, Sigmund, 70
Friedman, Dr. Henry, 29-30, 33, 36-37,
    41, 48, 116, 193-194, 244
frontal lobotomy, 111
fruits, antioxidant-rich, 211
fumagillin, 78
funding, 72, 82, 94, 115, 176, 190,
    234, 236

gadolinium, 15, 73, 75
galactoside, 199
gamma-interferon, 213, 215
gamma-linolenic acid (GLA), 57-58, 62,
    87-88, 93, 101, 113, 117, 162, 202,
    217-221, 224, 230, 240; mechanism
    of action, 88, 219, 221; side effects of,
    57, 99
garlic, 211, 224
gene therapy, 40-41, 246-248, 254
genetic(s), 4, 122, 155-156, 241, 246-
    249; mutations, 86, 207, 210, 218,
    231, 239, 241
genistein, 221-225, 231, 240, 243;
    mechanism of action, 223
Germany, 180
ginger, 211
ginseng, 176, 211
Glass, Dr. Jon, 92, 94, 133, 252
Gleevec (STI-571), 138-139, 243
Gliadel, 125-127, 132, 154; side effects
    of, 132

glioblastoma multiforme (GBM), 1, 11,
    13, 15, 17, 19, 21, 23, 25-27, 33-34,
    43-46, 51, 54, 62-64, 66-67, 76, 85-
    87, 89, 91-94, 98, 101, 104, 109, 112,
    114-115, 117, 119-120, 125-128,
    132-133, 136, 151, 154-157, 164-
    165, 175, 193, 195, 197, 213-214,
    216-217, 220, 222, 229, 231, 236,
    242-245, 248-252, 254
gliomas, 22, 26, 29, 33, 44-45, 47-48,
    56-57, 62, 67, 87-88, 92, 94, 98-100,
    105, 120, 125, 126, 128-129, 131-
    133, 141, 155, 158-159, 181, 184,
    195, 199-200, 216, 219, 223-224,
    230-231, 243, 244, 252, 254-255
glucosamine, 177
glucose, 179
glutathione, 208, 226. See also antioxidants.
glycoprotein, 254
Gold, Dr. Joseph, 143, 172, 179-180,
    197-198
grandfather clause, 126, 128
granulocyte-macrophage colony-stimulat-
    ing factor (GM-CSF), 252
Great Britain, 99-100, 125, 132, 159,
    219-220, 228
green tea, 176, 202, 222, 225, 240
Green, Saul, 176, 191, 202, 222, 225, 240
growth factors, 88, 93, 139, 223, 231,
    237, 241-244, 246, 249, 251-255
Gruber, Dr. Michael, 92

Hahnemann University, 242
Harvard Medical School, 7-8, 25, 91, 93,
    102-103, 236
hawthorn fruit, 211
head and neck cancer, 139
heart disease, 7, 143, 176, 207, 217
helplessness, sense of, 96-97
hematocrit, 254
hemoglobin, 66
Henry Ford Hospital, 38
hepatoma, 200
HER2 oncogene, 246, 254
herbal treatments, 173, 176, 185, 200-201
Herceptin, 245-246, 254

herpes virus, 40-41, 247, 254
Herrnstein, Richard, 7, 43
high-intensity brachytherapy, 39
Hippocrates, 133
Hippocratic oath, 130, 133, 165, 186
histology slides, 29, 244
historical controls, 152-154, 158-159, 210
HIV, 86-87, 238, 249
HMO, 30, 78-81
Hodgens, Dr. David, 101
Hodgkin's disease, 119, 233
holistic medicine, 172-173, 199. *See also* alternative medicine.
homeopathy, 172. *See also* alternative medicine.
hope, 2, 27, 96, 129
hormones, 54, 199, 212-213, 229
hospice care, 102
Human Genome Project, 247
Huxley, Aldous, 43
Hydergine, 204
hydration, 194
hydrazine sulfate, 179-180, 196, 198-199
hydroxyl radicals, 213
hypertension, 46, 199

ibuprofen, 218
ImClone Systems Incorporated, 139, 143, 254
immune system, 140, 184, 212-213, 218, 243, 247, 249-250, 252; boosting, 33, 54, 88, 172-174, 181-182, 215, 249; suppressed, 199, 203, 249
Immunocal, 226
immunological detection, of foreign proteins, 249, 251
immunotherapy, 250-251, 255
impairment, 4, 22, 63-64
ImuVert, 184
in vitro studies, 57, 62, 182, 200, 215, 224, 231
India, 56-57, 99, 113, 217, 219
infection, 7, 101, 216, 243; postsurgical, 21, 184
inflamed lungs, 55, 65-66, 68
inflammation, 66, 250

inflammatory agents, 181, 218, 236, 243, 250
inflammatory cytokines, 236
infusion procedure, for treating brain tumors, 41, 234, 239, 251
insurance, 51, 190, 215
intellect, 1
intensive care, 19-20
interleukin receptors, 243
interleukin-1 (IL-1), 213
interleukin-2 (IL-2), 213-215, 229, 250-251, 255
interleukin-4 (IL-4), 243, 252
interleukin-13 (IL-13), 243
interleukins, 213-215, 229, 243, 250-252, 255
internal capsule, 13, 38
Internet, 2, 29, 31, 51, 65, 98, 100, 116, 118, 163, 165, 257-258
internists, 12, 14, 18, 47
Interstate Commerce Act, 189
intracranial catheter, 243, 250
Investigational New Drug (IND) permit, 188, 190
iodine seeds, radioactive, 34, 38, 40, 123, 242, 245
iron, 35, 219. *See also* pro-oxidants.
Iscador, 180-182, 196, 199
iscumen, 181
isomer, 221
isotretinoin, 51, 115, 243
Italy, 54, 99, 113, 213, 244

Japan, 28, 54, 66, 93, 215, 217, 225
journals, medical, 43-44, 62, 105, 131-132, 143, 159, 175, 191, 198-200, 204, 210, 228-231, 252-255

Kaposi's sarcoma, 91, 141, 236
Karnofsky score, 122, 149, 152, 155-158
Kefauver, Senator Carey Estes, 142
killer cell activity, 213, 250, 255
kindling, 32
Kormanik, Patricia, 25, 52, 66, 79, 81
krestin, 54-55, 88, 93, 162, 215-216, 224, 229-230

Kytril, 49

lactic acid, 179
laetrile, 178-179, 196
leaks, 211
lectins, 181
lentils, 211
lentinan, 215-217
leprosy, 116, 141, 236
lesions, 14
leukemia, 7, 175, 216, 225, 243;
    childhood, 87, 119, 233; chronic
    myelogenous, 138
leukocyte, 181
Levin, Dr. Victor, 51, 62, 115-116
libido, loss of, 68, 76, 185
library, medical school, 27, 31, 65, 204
licorice root, 211
life expectancy, 71, 241. *See also*
    survival rate.
Life Extension Foundation, The, 204-
    205, 222, 227, 258
life-and-death decisions, 75, 146
life-threatening disease, 1-4, 7-8, 12, 14,
    16, 18, 20, 22, 24, 26-28, 30, 32, 34,
    36, 38, 40, 42, 44, 46, 48-50, 52-54,
    56, 58-60, 62-64, 66, 68, 70, 72, 74,
    76-78, 80, 82, 86, 88, 90, 92, 94-98,
    100, 102, 110, 112, 114-116, 118,
    120, 122, 124, 126, 128, 130-134,
    136-138, 140, 142, 146, 148, 150,
    152, 154, 156, 158, 161-162, 164-
    166, 172, 174, 176, 178, 180, 182,
    184, 186, 188, 190, 192, 194, 196-
    198, 200, 202, 204, 206, 208-210,
    212, 214, 216, 218, 220, 222, 224,
    226-228, 230, 232, 234, 236, 238,
    240-244, 246, 248, 250, 252, 254,
    258, 260
lifestyle changes, 7, 173-174, 209, 233
limonene, 225
linoleic acid, 217, 221
lipoic acid, 208
liver, 203, 240, 253
liver cancer, 214, 216, 225
liver toxicity, 36, 51, 76, 115, 120

lobotomy, 111
localized treatment, 34, 41, 76, 245
Loeffler, Dr. Jay, 101-102
lomustine, 41
long-term survivors, 2, 28, 95, 97-100,
    105, 109, 157, 175, 258
lovastatin, 225
low-intensity brachytherapy, 39, 222
lungs, inflamed, 55, 65-66, 68
lung cancer, 7, 43, 62, 140, 142-143,
    183, 198-199, 208-211, 214, 216,
    222, 224-225, 228-230, 233-234
lupus, 141, 208, 237
lycopene, 212, 229
lymph nodes, 7, 229, 251
lymphocyte killer cells, 250
lymphokine, 255

M.D. Anderson Cancer Center, 51, 115-
    116, 158, 176, 248
macrobiotic diet, 20, 174
macular degeneration, 76
magnetic resonance imaging (MRI),
    15-17, 21-24, 29, 36-37, 47, 52-54,
    56, 58-61, 65-68, 71-81, 85, 95,
    116, 194
maitake, 216
maitake D-fraction, 216, 230
malignancy, 1, 20, 39, 44-45, 62, 79, 85,
    89, 120, 131-133, 139, 156, 159, 200,
    212, 219, 223, 229-230, 235, 242-
    243, 248, 254-255
malnourished, 220
Mann-Whitney U., 158
marijuana, 48-49, 62
marimastat, 90, 154
Marshall, Dr. Larry, 18, 20-22, 25, 34-
    38, 40-41, 48, 57-58, 62, 79-81, 95-
    96, 101
Mayo Clinic Cancer Center, 178, 193,
    206, 208
median survival times, 39, 45-46, 54, 92,
    95, 124-126, 129, 150-151, 164, 181,
    183, 193, 195, 211, 220, 236, 242,
    248, 250
medical errors, 49, 112, 148

meditation, 174

Medscape, 259

melanoma, 181, 183, 185, 199-200, 213-214, 221-222, 224, 233, 249, 251

melatonin, 54, 87-88, 93, 99, 212-214, 249; effects on immune system, 54, 88, 212-213; mechanism of action, 54, 88; side effects of, 54, 87, 93, 99, 212-214, 249

memory, 70, 75

meningitis, 102

meta-analysis, 132

metabolic rate, 207, 221

metabolism, 173, 179, 182, 207-208, 217, 219

metalloproteinase inhibitors (MMPIs), 89-90

metastatic tumors, 91, 97, 119, 174, 181, 183, 197-199, 214-216, 223-224, 229, 231, 238, 241, 246, 254

Mexico, 42, 51, 116

microscopic tumor cells, 22, 67, 77

midbrain, 38, 58

milk thistle, 240

mind-body interactions, 199

minerals, 173, 201

mistletoe, 176, 180, 199

Mitchell, Dr. Malcolm, 39

Moniz, Dr. Antonio, 111

monoclonal antibodies (MABs), 29, 33, 36-37, 41, 48, 53, 116, 139-140, 223, 242, 244-246, 251-252, 254

monoterpenes, 225

monounsaturated fatty acids, 217

mortality rates, 43, 198, 209, 235

Moss, Dr. Ralph, 178

motor function tests, 20

motor tract, 13, 38, 40, 58

multiple drug approach. *See* drug cocktails.

Multiple Regression Analysis, 158

multiple sclerosis, 12-13

mung beans, 211

Musella, Al, 105, 258

mushroom extracts, 54-55, 88, 93, 162, 165, 181, 211, 215-217, 224, 229-230, 249

mutation, cellular, 86, 207, 231, 237, 239

myelinated nerve fibers, 75, 83

myeloma, 141, 236

narcotic, 21

National Academy of Sciences, 26, 227-228, 232

National Cancer Institute (NCI), 91, 113, 143, 153, 176, 180, 182, 187, 192-193, 239, 252, 254

National Institutes of Health (NIH), 72, 78, 191, 193, 204, 206, 225, 228, 258

National Science Foundation, 72

naturopath, 172

nausea, 19-20, 30, 48-49, 119

necrotic tissue, 38-39

neural tissue, 1, 83

neuro-oncologist, 18, 25, 29, 35, 39, 43-45, 51, 54, 57, 67, 79-80, 87-88, 93, 99, 109-110, 115-117, 127-129, 153, 158, 164, 193, 231

neuroblastoma, 225

neurohormone, 213

neurological deficits, 25

neurological dysfunction, 12

neurological symptoms, 39, 68

neurologist, 13, 15, 79-80, 95, 97, 136, 229

neuropil, 41

neuroscience, 13, 32, 79

neurosurgeon, 13, 18, 22, 35, 39, 48, 79-81, 101, 110, 136, 219

neutropenic, 59

New York Medical College, 77

New York University, 92

Newcastle disease, 184-185, 200

nitrosoureas, 48, 62, 105, 125. *See also* ACNU, BCNU, CCNU.

Nixon, Richard, 233-234

node-relapsed melanoma, 214

non-small cell lung cancer, 198-199, 211, 214, 216, 228-230

nonparametric statistics, 158

nontoxic agents, 51, 57, 115, 137-138, 162, 164, 166, 202-203, 241, 250

Novartis Pharmaceuticals, 248
null hypothesis, 124, 147-148, 154
numbness, 2, 11, 20, 37, 45, 56, 68, 70-71, 79, 82, 99, 109, 113-114, 119, 122, 127, 129, 132, 150, 152-153, 158, 169, 177, 179, 181-185, 190, 192, 195, 203, 206, 208-209, 211, 214, 223, 235-236, 242, 251, 257
nutriceuticals, 201, 217
nutrition, 204, 210, 228-229, 231, 253
nutritional supplements. *See* supplements.

obesity, 209
occipital cortex, 58
off-label usage, 117, 141
Office of Alternative Medicine, 191
Oldfield, Dr. Edward, 40
oleander, 176
oleic acid, 231
oligoastrocytoma, 132
oligodendroglioma, 100
olives, 211
omega-3 fatty acids, 217-218, 230
omega-6 fatty acids, 217-218
oncogene, 246, 254
oncologist, 4, 28, 36, 52, 65, 80, 97, 101-104, 113-115, 117-118, 120-121, 126-127, 139, 142-143, 154, 161-163, 165, 167, 169, 173-176, 183, 191, 197, 209-210, 213, 217, 240, 257-258
oncology, 3-4, 43-44, 54, 62, 80, 89, 94, 110, 116, 131-133, 150, 156, 159, 162, 181, 198-200, 207, 213, 217, 228-231, 252, 254, 258-259
oncolysate, 200
onions, 211, 224-225
Online Secrets of Top Health and Medical Researchers, The, 257
ovarian cancer, 214, 225, 231, 234, 253-254
oxidation, 207-208

p53 tumor suppressor gene, 210, 219
Packer, Dr. Lester, 207-208, 228
pain, 3, 21, 25, 42, 50, 68; controlling, 21

pancreatic cancer, 99, 139, 176, 183, 197, 200, 214, 220, 225, 230
paralysis, 38, 64
parietal cortex, 13-14, 38, 58, 63-64
parsley, 211
partial response, to treatment, 54, 193
pathology report, 25
patient characteristics, 4, 32, 122, 147, 149, 151-152, 155, 209, 246
patient population, 112, 148, 153, 206
patient profile, 122, 146, 152-153, 155, 161, 172
patient-specific vaccine, 251
patients' rights, 3, 156
Pauling, Dr. Linus, 206, 227-228
PCV, 25, 41, 48, 53, 55-56, 58, 62, 65, 67-68, 132, 195; side effects of, 58
perilla oil, 217
perillyl alcohol, 225
personality, 1, 8, 81, 110
pharmacists, 49
phenothiazine, 46
physical stamina, 64, 68
Physician's Desk Reference (PDR), 49, 120
phytic acid, 227
pineal gland, 54, 212, 229
placebo, 44, 90, 112, 125-127, 131, 151, 154, 175, 180, 184, 198-199, 209, 220, 224, 230
placebo effect, 111, 119
platelet count, 214
platelet-derived growth factor, 237
platinum drugs, 47, 113, 119
Poly ICLC, 33, 51, 153-154, 195, 249
polymer wafers, 125
polyphenolic catechins, 225
polyps, intestinal, 205
polysaccharide krestin (PSK), 55, 88, 93, 162, 215-216, 224, 229-230; mechanism of action, 54, 88
polysaccharides, 181, 216, 230
polyunsaturated fatty acids, 162, 217, 230-231. *See also* gamma-linolenic acid.
postsurgical problems, 21
prescription, 34, 41-42, 47, 49, 51, 116, 120, 130, 141, 213, 236, 240-241

pressure, intracranial, 21, 194, 243
primrose oil, 57, 220
pro-oxidants, 219
probabilistic treatment effects, 4, 109, 151, 164-165
probability levels, statistical, 4, 76, 86, 110, 123-124, 126, 140, 147-148, 151, 153, 157-158
probability, laws of, 86, 110
procarbazine, 48, 55, 62, 68, 87, 125-126, 132; side effects of, 56
professional antigen-presented cells, 251
prognosis, 1-2, 20, 25-27, 31, 42, 62, 69, 72, 96, 109, 140, 155, 159, 175, 183-184, 194, 198, 210, 227, 234, 244, 249
prognostic indicators, 104, 109, 122, 149
promising treatments, 4, 41, 57, 64, 75, 92, 113, 118, 121, 123-125, 127-131, 133, 135, 140, 142-143, 147-148, 150, 156, 161, 176, 185, 196, 203, 225, 234
prostaglandin, 218, 253
prostate cancer, 91, 174-175, 185, 200, 209, 211-214, 218, 221, 224, 231, 234-236, 253
protein kinase C, 33, 88, 93, 219, 223, 243
protein, 28, 181, 203, 213, 217-218, 225, 231
proteinase, 89
PSA levels, 185, 212, 234
Pseudomonas, 243
psychological impact, of cancer, 96-97, 199
PubMed, 31, 258
pulmonary fibrosis, 66
pulmonary metastases, 224
pulmonary problems, 55, 65-66, 68, 224

Q10, 202, 208, 227
Quackwatch, 177-178, 180-181, 184, 191, 193, 198
quality of life, 64, 146, 175, 180, 214
quercetin, 225, 231

radiation oncologist, 28, 101
radiation treatment, 22, 25-30, 32, 34, 36-39, 43-46, 62, 74-75, 87, 93, 101-

102, 104, 109, 119, 122, 127, 129, 131-132, 139-140, 146, 155, 157, 159, 175, 181, 183, 194, 197, 199, 206, 209-210, 214, 219, 230, 240, 242, 244-245, 253; whole-head, 101. *See also* DNA damage
radioactive iodine, 34, 38, 40, 123, 242, 245
radiologist, 52, 73-74
radiosurgery, 75-76, 127, 146
randomized clinical trial, 44, 131-132, 136, 138, 153, 155, 180, 183-184, 198-199, 209, 212-215, 224, 229-231
recombinant adenovirus, 249
recombinant DNA, 238, 248-249, 254
recovery, 15, 19, 21, 36, 59, 65, 68, 72, 102
recurrence, tumor, 27, 33, 39-40, 44, 66-67, 71-72, 75-78, 85-86, 89, 91-92, 94, 120, 125, 129, 131-133, 140, 146, 159, 184, 193, 200, 216, 236, 238, 248, 250, 252, 254-255
red meat, 202, 221
reishi, 216
relapse, 128, 132, 229
remission, 56, 66, 77, 225
reproductive system, 213
residual tumor, 22, 30, 37-38, 40, 46, 48, 52-53, 56-58, 66-69, 71, 76-77, 80, 85, 92, 109, 194
Retin-A, 115
Revici's cancer protocol, 213
rheumatoid arthritis, 218, 230
risk, of undergoing treatment, 34, 38, 42, 46, 76, 88, 118, 120, 124, 131, 137, 142, 164, 174-175, 181, 185
rituximab, 254
Rose, Dr. Jed, 29
Rosenthal Center, 258
rosiglitazone, 240
Russia, 179, 239

Salazar, Dr., 33, 44
sarcoma, 91, 141, 181, 236
saturated fatty acids, 217
scallions, 211

scar tissue, 58-59, 194

schizophrenia, 46, 111, 166

Scripps Memorial Hospital, 30

Sehydrin, 198

seizure, 31-32, 96

selenium, 208, 224, 231

self-prescription, 120

Selker, Dr. Robert, 34, 42, 77, 133

senega root, 211

sensorimotor deficits, 97

Serratia marcescens, 184, 200

sesame seeds, 211

714X, 176, 184

shark cartilage, 176, 203, 205

shiitake mushrooms, 211, 215-216

silver fillings, 173

silymarin, 240, 253

skin cancer, 181, 183, 185, 199-200, 213-214, 221-222, 224, 233, 249, 251

sleep cycles, 212

Sloan-Kettering Cancer Center, 176, 178-179, 193

small cell lung cancer, 62, 140, 142, 210, 229

smoking, 29, 209, 233, 235

sodium levels, 44, 194

Southwest Neuro-Imaging Center, 192

soy products, 202, 211, 221-223, 231, 243

soybean oil, 217

Spence, Dr. Alexander, 39

SPES, 185, 211

squalamine, 253-254

squamous cell cancers, 242

St. John's wort, 177

stabilization, of disease, 92, 116, 129, 153, 226, 236, 239, 241, 246

standard treatment, 4, 35, 101, 103-104, 109, 117-118, 127-129, 131, 174, 183, 185, 211, 214-215, 246

staphylococcus, 251

statistical noise, 148-149, 157

statistical significance, 113, 121, 123-126, 142, 145, 147-151, 155, 157-158, 216

statistics, 25, 31, 95, 98, 109, 124, 158, 198; nonparametric, 158

Steiner, Rudolf, 180-181

steroids, 21, 194

STI-571 (Gleevec), 138-139, 243

stomach cancer, 216, 221

stomachache, 56, 68

stress, 97, 174, 199, 207-208, 228

success, of treatment, 1-2, 4, 28, 54, 77, 87, 98, 112, 115, 118-119, 128-129, 153, 172, 174, 176, 183, 191-192, 196-197, 234, 242-243, 245, 249

sugar pill. *See* placebo.

Sugiura, Dr. Kanematsu, 178

sulforaphane, 226

sulindac, 240, 253

sunflower oil, 221

supplements, 3, 66, 71, 120, 172-174, 176-177, 180, 185, 197, 201-207, 209, 211-213, 215, 217-225, 227, 229, 231, 258

surgery, 18-19, 21-22, 24-25, 27-32, 34-40, 46, 57-59, 69-71, 74, 81, 86, 95, 101, 109-110, 125, 136, 175, 194, 198, 212, 251

surgical complications, 21, 30, 59, 103

surgical scar, 26, 30, 58-59, 96, 194

survival, 1-2, 4, 8, 12, 14, 16, 18, 20, 22, 24, 26-28, 30, 32, 34, 36, 38, 40, 42, 44-62, 64-68, 70, 72, 74, 76, 78, 80, 82, 85-88, 92, 94-96, 98-100, 102, 109-110, 112, 114, 116, 118, 120, 122, 124, 126-130, 132, 134, 136-138, 140, 142-143, 146, 148, 150, 152, 154, 156-158, 162, 164, 166, 169, 172, 175-176, 178, 180, 182-184, 186, 188, 190, 192-194, 196, 198-200, 202, 204, 206, 208, 210-212, 214, 216, 218, 220, 222, 224, 226, 228, 230, 232, 234, 236-238, 240, 242, 244, 246, 248, 250, 252, 254-255, 258, 260; characteristics affecting, 122, 246

survival rate, 46, 48, 55, 66, 125-126, 129, 132, 157, 159, 164, 174-175, 183, 185, 198, 214, 216, 234-235l; for anaplastic astrocytoma patients, 45; for glioblastoma patients, 15, 22, 24, 27, 44-46, 54, 62, 66-67, 76, 92-94,

treatments, localized, 34, 41, 74, 76, 212, 245; marketing of, 49, 111-112, 117, 142, 156, 217, 222, 226; proven, 4, 113-114, 130, 138, 178, 189, 196; systemic, 75-76, 132, 255; unproven, 4, 109, 111, 114, 118, 127, 174, 189, 196

trial results, 28, 43-44, 54, 77-78, 112, 114, 117, 119, 122-124, 127, 136, 138, 147, 149, 151-152, 155-156, 159, 161, 164, 180, 189-190, 196, 211, 213, 236, 239, 248

trials, clinical, 28, 33, 39, 41-42, 44-45, 51, 55, 57, 64, 79, 90-92, 94, 98, 102-105, 109, 111-132, 135-143, 145-159, 161-164, 177-181, 183-186, 191-193, 195-196, 199-200, 202-205, 208-215, 219-220, 223-226, 228-231, 235-237, 239-244, 246-248, 251-252, 258

tumor cavity, 32, 52, 57, 99, 125, 217, 219, 244, 250

tumor necrosis factor, 237, 250

tumor, cancerous, 1, 9, 13-15, 17-20, 22, 24-30, 33, 35-40, 43-44, 48, 50-51, 53-59, 63-64, 66-67, 71-80, 86-90, 92-93, 96-101, 103-105, 109, 113, 116-119, 122-125, 128-132, 137, 146, 149, 152, 154-156, 158, 161, 171, 175, 184, 187, 192-195, 199-200, 203, 210-212, 214-217, 219, 221, 223-226, 228-229, 231, 235-239, 242-253, 255; defense mechanisms of, 46, 251; metastatic, 91, 97, 119, 174, 181, 183, 197-199, 214-216, 223-224, 229, 231, 238, 241, 246, 254; primary, 238; residual, 22, 30, 37-38, 40, 46, 48, 52-53, 56-58, 66-69, 71, 76-77, 80, 85, 92, 109, 194; visible, 22, 76

turmeric, 227

tyrosine kinase, 225, 231, 242-243, 246

Ukrain, 182-183, 196, 200

Unger, Dr. George, 187-188

University Hospital, San Diego, 25, 30

University of California, 11, 13, 18, 25, 27, 29, 31, 35, 39, 41, 46, 98, 102-103, 180

University of Michigan, 241

University of Pittsburgh, 34, 77

University of Southern California, 33

University of Vermont, 222

University of Washington, 39, 191

unmyelinated nerve fibers, 83

urinary infection, 21

urine, 187, 200, 238

vaccine, cancer, 184-185, 200, 251-252; generic, 251

vascular endothelial growth factor (VEGF), 237, 249, 253

vegetables, antioxidant-rich, 208-209, 211-212, 226, 232

verapamil, 47, 52, 55, 62; side effects of, 52

vinblastine, 199

vincristine, 48, 55, 62, 216; side effects of, 56, 68

Vioxx, 240

virus, 40-41, 82, 86, 185, 200, 247, 249, 254; immunological reaction to, 184, 247, 249

viscotoxin, 181

Viscum album, 199

visual cortex, 38

visual imaging, 174

vitamin A, 51-52, 208, 212; and cancer prevention, 115; high dosages of, 115, 208

vitamin B$_{17}$. *See* laetrile.

vitamin C, 183, 206-208, 228; and cancer prevention, 206

vitamin D$_3$, 240, 253

vitamin E, 30, 202, 207-210, 219-220, 228, 230

vitamins, 173-174, 201, 207-208, 228; mega-dosages of, 206, 208; supplements, 174, 185, 205-207, 212, 240. *See also* antioxidants and pro-oxidants.

Wales, 219

Walter Reed Hospital, 33

Printed in Great Britain
by Amazon

43019137R00167